PRINCIPLES OF MEASUREMENT
FOR ANAESTHETISTS

Principles of Measurement for Anaesthetists

M.K. SYKES

M.A. M.B. B.Chir.
D.A. F.F.A.R.C.S.
Professor of Clinical Anaesthesia,
Royal Postgraduate Medical School
Consultant Anaesthetist,
Hammersmith Hospital

M.D. VICKERS

M.B. B.S. M.R.C.S. L.R.C.P.
D.A. F.F.A.R.C.S.
Consultant Anaesthetist and
Consultant to the Department of
Clinical Investigation and Research
Dudley Road Hospital, Birmingham
Honorary Lecturer,
University of Birmingham

BLACKWELL SCIENTIFIC PUBLICATIONS

OXFORD AND EDINBURGH

SBN 632 06910 4

FIRST PUBLISHED 1970

Printed in Great Britain by
SPOTTISWOODE, BALLANTYNE & CO. LTD.
LONDON AND COLCHESTER
and bound by
THE KEMP HALL BINDERY
OXFORD

Contents

v

Contents

PART III
HANDLING NUMERICAL DATA

Preface

Ten years ago few anaesthetists measured anything more than respiration rate, pulse rate and blood pressure. Today the anaesthetist routinely uses a number of other measurements and is expected to understand the principles of many more. Two factors have been mainly responsible for this change in practice: first, the increased complexity of surgery, and in particular the advent of open-heart surgery, and secondly the refinement of techniques used in resuscitation and intensive care.

Nearly all the techniques of measurement now employed in clinical practice were originally developed by painstaking research in the laboratory. The original publications dealing with these techniques are often lengthy and detailed and the average anaesthetist has not the time, or inclination, to read them all. For this reason the authors have attempted to produce a short text which outlines the principles of all the physical methods of measurement likely to be encountered by the anaesthetist. Some of these techniques have, as yet, only a research application: these have been dealt with in principle. A certain number of techniques will be used by the anaesthetist during the course of his clinical work. Additional detail has been provided in these sections so that the anaesthetist is made aware of the main technical pitfalls likely to be encountered. Selected references provide a guide to further reading.

This book has been divided into three sections. The introductory section describes the physical principles used in measurement. The second section deals with specific types of measurement. The third section provides an outline of the statistical methods appropriate to the presentation and interpretation of the types of numerical data which are likely to be produced by the instruments discussed in this book. It is hoped that this arrangement will allow the text to be used both as a reference book and as a general introduction to the subject.

Books on this and related topics are usually written by experts with a deep knowledge of the field. This generally makes it difficult for them to provide a simple explanation without qualification. The authors of this book, after prolonged professional involvement in postgraduate education in anaesthesia, believe that this exalted approach may often be totally unproductive. They have not hesitated, therefore, to simplify whenever it was felt that it would assist comprehension. Nothing beyond the rudiments of 1st M.B. physics and O-level mathematics is assumed and every attempt has been made to avoid jargon, or, where it occurs, to explain its meaning.

It is hoped that this simple, if somewhat dogmatic, approach will enable anaesthetists and postgraduate students of anaesthesia to obtain a working knowledge of the physical principles of instrumentation in the shortest possible time.

April, 1970

M.K. SYKES
M.D. VICKERS

Introduction

The administration of an anaesthetic must always be governed by the patient's response to the anaesthetic drugs and to the surgical insult. This response is most simply assessed by observing the pattern of respiration, changes in the pulse and skin colour and the neurological reaction to the surgical stimulus. However, all these observations are open to subjective error and they are, therefore, usually supplemented by certain objective measurements such as blood pressure, pulse rate and minute volume. Unfortunately, these measurements only provide a rough guide to the condition of the patient, for they are not directly related to the basic functions which should be measured. Blood pressure, for example, depends on both cardiac output and peripheral resistance, whilst minute volume is but one of several factors affecting arterial Pco_2. In clinical practice it is now essential that the anaesthetist should know, not only that blood pressure is low, but why it is low. Furthermore, he must not only be capable of diagnosing and treating abnormalities of function but he must also be capable of preventing such changes by providing a normal biological environment for the cell. In short, the anaesthetist has now become a clinical physiologist as well as a clinical pharmacologist, and techniques of measurement are now an integral part of his daily life.

The first essential in the making of any measurement is that the operator should understand the principle on which the measurement is based and should know the degree of specificity which may be expected. Failure to observe this seemingly simple requirement has resulted in many analytical errors in the past when, for example, a breakdown product has been measured instead of the original agent. The second essential is that the measurement must be referred to an internationally agreed standard, so that the units of measurement are comparable. The third essential is that the accuracy of the measurement must be known, not only in terms of the accuracy possible with a given instrument, but also in terms of the accuracy obtained in the hands of the user. The last essential is that the normal range of the measurement should be established so that its biological significance can be correctly assessed.

This book deals mainly with the first two requirements, namely the principles of measurement and the standards by which such measurements are judged. The third requirement, accuracy, depends largely on the choice of method, available instrumentation and the ability of the user: it can therefore only be discussed in general terms. The last requirement, the establishment of a normal range of values, is more properly the province of physiologists and clinicians and the reader is referred to other texts for information on the interpretation of the measurements herein described.

Finally, a word of warning. Instruments look impressive and often produce intriguing information. However, the results obtained from an instrument are only as good as the person who operates it; often they are much worse. It is therefore essential that an instrument should only be used to confirm or extend our clinical observation of the patient. It will be many years before instrumentation systems can match the efficiency of the human brain in the perception and interpretation of the many signals which continually bombard our senses. When this stage is reached this book will no longer be necessary.

Part 1
General Principles
of Measurement

1
Principles of Measurement

Successful medical treatment depends on accurate diagnosis. Diagnosis is, in turn, based on the history and on the elicitation of physical signs. Simple instruments, such as the stethoscope, facilitate the detection of such signs. Other instruments, such as the thermometer, increase the accuracy with which changes can be measured. More complicated instruments, such as the electrocardiograph, enable changes outside the range of human perception to be charted.

Instruments are therefore used in medicine either to display or record signals which can be appreciated by the human senses, or to detect, display and record signals which are outside the range of human perception. In either event the system must consist of a detector, which senses the signal, and some form of display. The signal may be transferred directly from detector to display or may be altered in some way to make it more suitable for display. Finally the signal may be used to actuate a warning device, or even to set in motion a mechanism which reacts back upon the patient and controls some aspect of function. This plan is summarised below:

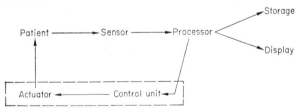

Sensing devices
Signals may originate from physical or physico-chemical changes within the body.

Physical. The source of energy may be heat, light, sound,

3

electricity, or it may be mechanical (force or movement). A movement may be transmitted directly to a display or recorder by a thread or lever: with other sources of energy it is usually necessary to convert the source energy into some other form of energy (e.g. electrical) which is more suitable for transmission or processing. A device which senses one source of energy and changes it into another form of energy is known as a transducer. Transducers are used for such measurements as pressure, displacement, temperature and flow.

Certain aspects of bodily function (nerve or muscle activity) are accompanied by electrical activity which can be sensed by electrodes placed on the active tissue or situated more remotely on the body surface. One of the difficulties in recording from such sites is that electrodes tend to develop a high resistance (become polarised) when placed in tissues. In the case of remote electrodes, there is a high skin resistance to be overcome. Since the changes in potential are usually small (of the order of millivolts) such resistances must be minimised if satisfactory recordings are to be obtained.

Physico-chemical. Many physico-chemical changes are examined by sending specimens to the laboratory for analysis. However, the increasing use of electrometric methods for the measurement of Po_2, Pco_2 and pH has finally led to the development of electrodes which can be inserted directly into the circulation or into an exteriorised loop of the circulation. This enables a continuous record to be obtained. In this situation the electrodes function as transducers and convert a change in gas tension or pH into electrical energy. A photo-electric cell may be used similarly to sense the intensity of light of a particular wavelength transmitted through a thin layer of blood. This type of sensor may be applied to the ear and used to record changes in O_2 saturation, or changes in dye concentrations in the determination of cardiac output.

Processing devices

In a few situations the signal can be transmitted directly to the recorder or display unit without intermediate processing. An obvious example of this is the sensing of pressure by a tambour, the latter being connected by a thread to a lever writing on a smoked drum. Usually, however, the signal from the electrode or transducer is inadequate to drive a display or recorder. The signal must, accordingly, be amplified before transmission. This can sometimes be accomplished mechanically, but is more commonly carried out by changing the signal into electrical energy first. This energy can then be amplified to a degree which would be quite impossible by the use of mechanical methods. Most processing units are more complex and modify the signal in some other way. For example, a flow signal from a pneumotachograph may be integrated to give a signal proportional to volume; impulses from a nerve fibre may be counted, and their frequency displayed; or an alinear output from a rapid gas analyser may be rendered linear before being displayed or recorded.

Display
The design of data display units has been sadly neglected in the past. As the volume of data increases and the time allowed for digestion of the data decreases (e.g. in aviation), display has been subjected to closer study. Unfortunately, progress in methods of display has only been slowly assimilated into the medical field.

Information may be displayed numerically as a digital display, on a scale, by graphical methods, or by other systems such as lights of varying intensity, colour and size. The method chosen should communicate the information clearly and with a minimum of distracting detail. The scale should be easily visible and safety limits (if any) clearly demarcated.

Meters. The mechanism most commonly employed in display systems is the moving-coil galvanometer. This consists of a coil of wire suspended on a thin wire or thread in a magnetic field (Fig. 1.1). When a current is passed through the coil a force is generated which rotates the coil against the torsion of the thread. The degree of rotation of the coil is then displayed by the movement of a needle attached to the coil. Since meters are usually used for the display of slowly changing signals, the mass of the coil and needle is not critical and a large coil can be used to increase sensitivity. However, when the moving-coil galvanometer is used for photographic recording much smaller coils are used to facilitate a rapid response and sensitivity is reduced.

The movement of the coil may also be displayed by shining a narrow beam of light onto a small mirror attached to the coil. The reflected beam is then directed onto a translucent scale. The use of a mirror greatly reduces the mass of the moving parts of the instrument and so increases the frequency response. Furthermore, by increasing the length of the light path (usually by a

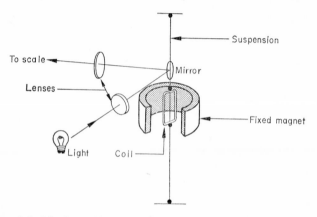

FIG. 1.1. Moving-coil galvanometer utilising a light source and mirror.

system of fixed mirrors), it is possible to increase the sensitivity of the system. Mirror galvanometers are therefore commonly used when it is desired to obtain maximum sensitivity and speed of response. They are also used in photographic recorders. (See Chapter 4.)

Traces or graphical plots. These are most conveniently displayed on a cathode-ray oscilloscope (Fig. 1.2). In this instrument a beam of electrons is generated (at the cathode) and focused by a number of positively charged plates (anodes) so that it appears as a small spot of light on the fluorescent screen. The characteristics of this screen can be chosen to provide the most appropriate duration of fluorescence. The beam of electrons can be deflected in the horizontal axis by applying a potential to one pair of plates, generally referred to as the X-plates, or deflected vertically by applying a potential to the Y-plates. (These are so called because they correspond to the conventional designations on the axes of graphs.) Normally, a potential derived from a special time-base circuit is applied to the X-plates. This potential gradually increases to a maximum and then suddenly returns to zero. The spot is thus moved steadily across the screen from left to right and rapidly returned to the zero point. The

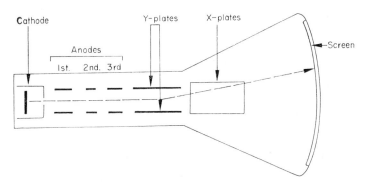

Fig. 1.2. Cathode-ray oscilloscope.

impression of a continuous trace is thus created. The signal to be recorded is usually applied to the Y-plates. In some applications two different signals are applied to the X and Y plates; a graphical plot then results. This method is often used to display pressure-volume loops in the study of lung mechanics. Vector-cardiography also utilises this kind of display.

Continuous traces can also be displayed on direct-writing or ultra-violet light recorders.

Digital display. This form of display is most suitable when the information is required in the form of figures, e.g. counts of nerve impulses, radioactivity, etc. The figures may be shown by special neon tubes or by direct print-out on paper. Obviously, the number of digits available must cover the range and accuracy required. This type of display eliminates errors due to faulty scale reading, but may introduce others, for example, in the position of the decimal point.

Recorders

Recorders may be broadly classified as direct-writing, photographic, and magnetic. In the first type a writing arm inscribes the signal directly on the paper. In the second type a display is photographed or a trace is recorded by moving a light spot across light sensitive paper or film. In the third type signals are recorded on magnetic tape or in a computer 'store' for subsequent play-back or re-recording. Recorders are dealt with more fully in Chapter 4.

Control devices

Control devices are used most frequently to achieve automation in industry. Their use in medicine has been restricted mainly to experimental applications since technical failure would often have serious consequences. A number of control devices have been produced for use in anaesthesia. Frumin (1957) produced a servo-ventilator in which ventilation was automatically adjusted in response to the end-tidal P_{CO_2}. This has been further developed so that if the patient breathes spontaneously a further dose of suxamethonium will be administered! Before this Kiersey, Faulconer & Bickford (1954) had developed a control device which regulated the depth of thiopentone anaesthesia on the basis of the E.E.G. More recent devices include one which switches on a pacemaker when the heart rate slows below a predetermined level and another which regulates the temperature of an incubator to maintain a constant abdominal skin temperature in neonates.

ESSENTIAL REQUIREMENTS OF
INSTRUMENTATION SYSTEMS

Signal/noise ratio

When attempting to construct an instrumentation system it must first be decided whether it is possible to isolate the desired signal. Difficulties arise when the signal is hidden amongst other signals of like nature and the intensity of the signal is not greatly different from the intensity of the background. Since the background signals are usually of varying intensity and frequency, they produce a noise, rather than a pure note, when amplified and reproduced through a loudspeaker system. The first requirement of successful instrumentation is therefore that the signal/noise ratio should be high, i.e. that the signal should stand out

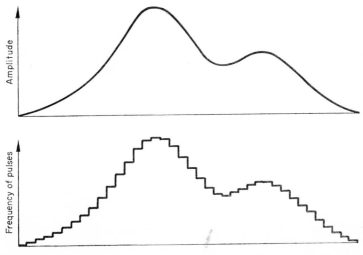

FIG. 1.3. Analogue to digital conversion.

clearly from the other signals which are likely to be picked up. Signal/noise ratio can often be improved by filtering out the unwanted frequencies electronically or by reinforcing the signal. An example of the latter technique is afforded by the C.A.T. (Computer of Average Transients). This can be used to reinforce any signal which recurs at a fixed interval. The input signal is first converted into a series of discrete pulses in such a manner that the number of pulses at each time interval represents the amplitude of the signal at that point. This is termed an analogue to digital conversion, and may be represented by the histogram in Fig. 1.3. The output from the converter is then fed into a series of magnetic cores, the electronic switching being so arranged that each group of impulses is fed into a separate core (Fig. 1.4). The sweep is initiated by a timing circuit or by triggering the switching circuit from some part of the recorded waveform. In other applications (e.g. evoked cortical responses from peripheral stimuli) the sweep may be triggered from the stimulator itself. If the sweep is now allowed to pass repeatedly over the magnetic cores there will be a gradual build-up of recorded impulses in

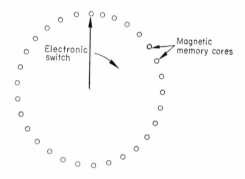

Fig. 1.4. Principle of a C.A.T. (Computer of Average Transients). The electronic switch makes contact with each of the cores in turn. Signals due to noise are deposited randomly amongst the cores, whereas a repetitive signal occurring at a fixed time interval after the start of each sweep builds up in a limited number of cores and is accentuated by each successive sweep.

each core. All of the cores will receive random pulses from the noise present in the signal, but the strength of signal in each core from this source will tend to average out at the same level in each core. However, in cores which receive the impulses originating from the repetitive signal the strength of the signal will build up at a much faster rate. This signal is therefore reinforced with each subsequent sweep and, on playback, the signal (which may have been concealed completely by the noise) now becomes obvious.

Repetitive signals may also be reinforced by using a time

exposure when photographing the display on an oscilloscope screen. Random variations in the waveform due to noise are averaged out across the film, whilst the path traced by the signal is reinforced at each successive sweep. In this way the image is caused to stand out from the background.

Accurate reproduction of input signal

The second requirement of any system of instrumentation is that it should provide an accurate display or record of the input signal. Most instrumentation systems are inherently unstable, their performance being affected by temperature, mains voltage and frequency, ageing of components, etc. When considering the accuracy of any system one must consider the zero stability, the gain stability, the linearity and frequency response. The latter includes a consideration of damping and phase shift.

Zero stability. The first aspect to be assessed is zero stability— the ability to maintain a zero reading on display or recorder when the input signal is zero. A certain amount of zero instability can usually be tolerated, but, obviously, the degree of stability required will vary with the application. For example, slight zero instability will prove less of a disadvantage when recording blood pressures during cardiac catheterisation than when recording blood pressures over prolonged periods of days or weeks.

Gain stability. The sensitivity of the processing device can usually be adjusted to vary the ratio between input and output signals by means of one or more 'gain' controls. There should always be ample reserve gain in the instrument and, once set, the degree of gain should remain constant over a period which is adequate for the purpose in hand.

Linearity. The degree of amplification of the signal should be equal throughout the whole range of signal strengths likely to be encountered. If this is not so the system is said to be alinear. Figure 1.5 illustrates alinearity in a blood pressure transducer–amplifier–recorder system which occurred only in the higher ranges of pressure.

Normally the linearity of an instrument or system is specified as being 'better than 1 per cent'. This means that the reading on the display unit should never be in error by more than ±1 per cent of the actual reading throughout the range of the instrument. Unfortunately, this statement sometimes only applies to part of the range and it is often difficult to determine the instrument's performance from the literature provided by the manufacturer. It is most important to assess the linearity of the complete system, since minimal alinearity in each component may prove additive and so lead to greater alinearity in the recorded signal.

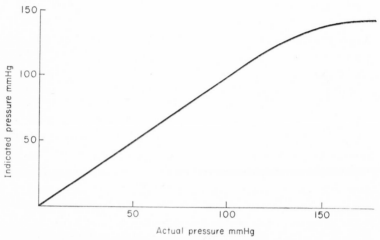

FIG. 1.5. Alinearity in a blood-pressure measuring system in the higher ranges of pressure.

Frequency response. Most signals follow a complicated pattern or waveform. Fourier showed that any complex waveform could be constructed by taking a simple sine wave of the same frequency as the slowest component (called the fundamental frequency) and adding to it a number of sine waves, the frequency of which bore a simple whole-number relationship to the fundamental. These higher-frequency waves are called harmonics of the fundamental frequency. Electrical and mechanical systems which transmit waveforms in fact behave as though all the components of a complex wave were really separate. To reproduce a complex wave accurately, therefore, the system must be able to handle all the components of the wave equally. This necessitates equal amplification of each component and, if any delay occurs in the system, there must be no alteration in the relative positions of the various components of the wave. Fortunately, it is unnecessary, as well as difficult, to adhere to the ideal solution, and for most practical purposes it is sufficient if the system reproduces accurately up to the tenth harmonic, that is, to ten times the fundamental frequency. For a pulse rate of 120/min (2 Hz), therefore, a flat response up to a frequency of 20 Hz is required for recording the blood-pressure wave. However, if one is particularly concerned with the high-frequency components, for example, when recording the rate of rise of a ventricular pressure trace, then a higher frequency response (40 Hz) would be necessary.

Matching. A complete instrumentation system consists of a number of components each of which has special characteristics. The efficiency of the complete system depends not only on the accuracy of the component parts but also the way they are matched to each other. Such matching must take account, not only of the strength and character of the signals fed from one component to another, but the way in which each component interacts with the other.

In complete systems this is properly taken care of by the maker, but when systems are constructed of separate 'black boxes' it is necessary to match both the current or voltage and the input and output impedances (see Chapter 3). If this is not done the characteristics of one part of the system may be considerably altered by the other. A false record may also be obtained by attaching a recorder to a device which normally feeds a meter. A recorder may shunt the meter, and provide a path for part of the signal. Both the recorder and the meter will then give a lower reading from a standard signal than would have been shown on the meter with the recorder unconnected.

It will be apparent from the above discussion that a large number of factors have to be taken into account when considering any system of measurement. Before a choice of instrumentation is made it is necessary to consider the degree of accuracy required and the manner in which the system is to be used. When these fundamentals have been decided detailed planning of the complete system becomes possible. If they are ignored the system may prove inadequate or unnecessarily expensive.

REFERENCES

FRUMIN M.J. (1957) Clinical use of a physiological respirator producing N_2O amnesia-analgesia. *Anesthesiology*, 18, 290.

KIERSEY D.K., FAULCONER A. & BICKFORD R.G. (1954) Automatic electro-encephalographic control of thiopental anesthesia. *Anesthesiology*, 15, 356.

FURTHER READING

GEDDES L.A. & BAKER L.E. (1968) *Principles of Applied Biomedical Instrumentation*. John Wiley & Sons, London.

LENIHAN J.M.A. (1969) *Instrumentation in Medicine*. Morgan-Grampian, London.

STOTT F.D. (1967) *Instruments in Clinical Medicine*. Blackwell Scientific Publications, Oxford and Edinburgh.

DEWHURST D.J. (1966) *Physical Instrumentation in Medicine and Biology*. Pergamon Press, Oxford.

HILL D.W. (1968) *Physics Applied to Anaesthesia*. Butterworth, London.

HILL, D.W. (1970) *Electronic Measurement Techniques in Anaesthesia and Surgery*. Butterworth, London.

CRUL J.F. and PAYNE J.P. (1970) *Patient monitoring*. Excepta Medica, Amsterdam.

2
Units of Measurement

Measurement became necessary when human beings began to exchange one commodity for another. Initially, measurements were related to commonly available objects. Thus in early Egyptian times length was related to the width of the finger (the digit) or to the distance from the elbow to the fingertips (the cubit). The fathom, equivalent to the 6-foot span of the arms, is still used for measuring the depth of the sea and the hand (4 inches) is still used for measuring the height of a horse. Later, an attempt was made to rationalise the measurements so that individual variation did not affect the comparisons. For example, the Egyptians standardised on the cubit and ordered that all other measurements should be fractions or multiples of a cubit. Thus the digit became one twenty-eighth of a cubit, and the fathom 4 cubits.

Even greater exactitude became possible when standards were adopted. Thus, even in Anglo-Saxon times, there was a standard yard, in the form of an iron bar kept at Winchester. A similar standard was maintained at Westminster until 1959, but after that date both the pound and the yard were related to the kilogramme and the metre.

Metric standards were first developed in France during the Revolution at the end of the 18th century. Initially the metre was supposed to be a distance equal to one ten-millionth of the distance along the earth's surface between the pole and equator, and the litre and kilogramme were defined from this primary standard. In 1875 an International Bureau of Weights and Measures was established at Sèvres, a suburb of Paris, and new standards of the metre and kilogramme were set up and sent to a number of countries. Later this International Bureau concerned itself with other standards. As the need for greater and greater accuracy has become apparent the Bureau has increasingly turned towards standards present in natural phenomena, since these can be measured by scientists anywhere in the world. Thus the standard metre (a bar made of platinum and iridium and kept at Sèvres) was dropped in 1960 in favour of a standard related to the wavelength of the orange light given off by Krypton-86 and, in 1967, time was related to atomic frequency.

Until 1960, therefore, there were two main systems of measurement in use in this country; the Imperial system was used for most purposes whilst the metric system was used in certain branches of science. Over the years, however, much time and thought have been expended in improving the metric system and, in 1960, the Conférence Générale des Poids et Mesures, the body responsible for maintaining standards of measurements, formally approved the S.I. system.

S.I. UNITS

S.I. is an abbreviation in many languages for Système International d'Unités, and is an extension and refinement of the traditional metric system. This system has now been adopted by a large number of countries and its use in the United Kingdom is being widely advocated. There are six basic S.I. units (Table 2.1).

It will be seen that the metre and kilogramme replace the

TABLE 2.1. Basic S.I. units.

Physical quantity	Name of unit	Symbol for unit*
Length	metre	m
Mass	kilogramme	kg
Time	second	s
Electric current	ampere	A
Thermodynamic temperature	degree Kelvin	°K
Luminous intensity	candela	cd

* Symbols for units do not take a plural form.

TABLE 2.2. Fractions and multiples.

Fraction	Prefix	Symbol	Multiple	Prefix	Symbol
10^{-1}	deci*	d	10	deka*	da
10^{-2}	centi*	c	10^2	hecto*	h
10^{-3}	milli	m	10^3	kilo	k
10^{-6}	micro	μ	10^6	mega	M
10^{-9}	nano	n	10^9	giga	G
10^{-12}	pico	p	10^{12}	tera	T

* It is hoped that these fractions and multiples will gradually cease to be used.

centimetre and gramme of the old metric system. It is also recommended that multiples of units should normally be restricted to steps of a thousand and fractions to steps of a thousandth (Table 2.2). Time continues to be measured in seconds, hours, days, etc. but the old electrostatic and electromagnetic units are replaced by S.I. electrical units. The unit of

TABLE 2.3. Supplementary units.

Physical quantity	Name of unit	Symbol for unit	Definition of unit
Energy	joule	J	$kg\ m^2\ s^{-2}$
Force	newton	N	$kg\ m\ s^{-2}$
Power	watt	W	$kg\ m^2\ s^{-3}$
Electric charge	coulomb	C	A s
Electric potential difference	volt	V	$kg\ m^2\ s^{-3}\ A^{-1}$
Electric resistance	ohm	Ω	$kg\ m^2\ s^{-3}\ A^{-2}$
Electric capacitance	farad	F	$A^2\ s^4\ kg^{-1}\ m^{-2}$
Magnetic flux	weber	Wb	$kg\ m^2\ s^{-2}\ A^{-1}$
Inductance	henry	H	$kg\ m^2\ s^{-2}\ A^{-2}$
Luminous flux	lumen	lm	cd sr
Illumination	lux	lx	$cd\ sr\ m^{-2}$
Frequency	hertz	Hz	cycle per second
Customary temperature	degree Celsius	°C	$t/°C = T/°K - 273\cdot15$
Plane angle	radian	rad $\left.\vphantom{\begin{matrix}a\\b\end{matrix}}\right\}$	have no dimensions
Solid angle	steradian	sr	

force is the *newton* (kilogramme metre per second per second) and the unit of energy in all forms is the *joule* (newton × metre). Power is measured in joules per second (watts) and the variously defined calories, B.t.u. and horsepower are all superseded. The names of some of these supplementary units are shown in Table 2.3 whilst a number of the derived units are illustrated in Table 2.4.

TABLE 2.4. Examples of other derived S.I. units.

Physical quantity	S.I. unit	Symbol for unit
Area	square metre	m^2
Volume	cubic metre	m^3
Density	kilogramme per cubic metre	$kg\ m^{-3}$
Velocity	metre per second	$m\ s^{-1}$
Angular velocity	radian per second	$rad\ s^{-1}$
Acceleration	metre per second squared	$m\ s^{-2}$
Pressure	newton per square metre	$N\ m^{-2}$
Kinematic viscosity, diffusion coefficient	square metre per second	$m^2\ s^{-1}$
Dynamic viscosity	newton second per square metre	$N\ s\ m^{-2}$
Electric field strength	volt per metre	$V\ m^{-1}$
Magnetic field strength	ampere per metre	$A\ m^{-1}$
Luminance	candela per square metre	$cd\ m^{-2}$

FUNDAMENTAL UNITS EMPLOYED
IN MECHANICS

The definitions of the units given in Tables 2.3 and 2.4 require some explanation. The reasoning can best be illustrated by considering some basic units employed in mechanics. The basic units are length (L), mass (M) and time (T) and in the S.I. system these units are the metre (m), kilogramme (kg) and second (s). Area, therefore, has the dimension of $L \times L = L^2$, and volume $= L^3$, so that the unit of area is the square metre (m^2) and the unit of volume is the cubic metre (m^3). Density is defined as mass per unit volume (M/L^3) so that the unit becomes kilogrammes per cubic metre (kg/m^3 or kg m^{-3}).

Velocity is defined as distance moved in unit time (L/T or LT^{-1}) and is therefore measured in metres per second (m/s or m s^{-1}), whilst acceleration is the rate of change of velocity, that is, metres per second per second (L/T^2 or m/s^2 or m s^{-2}). Force may be defined in terms of gravity or in absolute units. In the former system the force due to gravity acting on 1 kilogramme was termed the kilogramme force; it is now termed a kilopond. To define force in absolute units, advantage is taken of the fact that when a given mass is accelerated the acceleration produced is proportional to the force applied to the mass, i.e. force = mass × acceleration = ML/T^2 or kg m/s^2 or kg m s^{-2}. The force which will accelerate 1 kg at a rate of 1 metre per second per second is known as a newton.

Energy is the capacity to do work and therefore has the same units as work. It exists in two basic forms—potential energy (which results from the position of a body relative to surrounding bodies) and kinetic energy (which arises as a result of its motion). Energy is defined as force × distance moved = $ML/T^2 \times L$ = $ML^2 T^{-2}$, or in S.I. units kg m^2 s^{-2}.

Power is a function of force applied through a given distance in unit time (in other words, the rate at which work is done) and in S.I. units is 1 newton × 1 metre per second. This has the dimension of newton metres per second = kg m s^{-2} × m s^{-1} = kg m^2 s^{-3}.

Finally, pressure = force per unit area = MLT^{-2}/L^2 = $ML^{-1} T^{-2}$, or in S.I. units kg m^{-1} s^{-2} or newtons per square metre = N m^{-2}.

Similar reasoning can be applied to derive the other definitions given in Tables 2.3 and 2.4.

DEFINITIONS OF UNITS OF MEASUREMENT

The current standards are described in such publications as Documenta Geigy 'Scientific Tables' (7th Edition). The primary standards of a few commonly used units are detailed in Table 2.5.

TABLE 2.5. Methods used to define some common units of measurement.

Unit	Method
Metre	Vacuum wavelength of the orange-red spectral line of the atom of Krypton-86
Kilogramme	Mass of international prototype kilogramme (planimum–iridium cylinder kept at Sèvres, France)
Second	Atomic frequency of caesium-133
Electric current	Measure of the force between two parallel conductors created by the passage of a current
Thermodynamic temperature	1/273·16 of the thermodynamic temperature of the triple point of water (the point at which the solid, liquid and gaseous phases of pure water are in equilibrium)

THE TRANSITION TO S.I. UNITS

The adoption of new standards creates a number of difficulties which are not usually anticipated. When the standards are put into common use many of these difficulties disappear. A number of units of measurement based on the S.I. system are bound to prove inconvenient in some applications, and the S.I. system therefore makes allowance for the continuing use of some units which are at variance with the new proposals. Until the new system is thoroughly understood some duplication of units may prove desirable. Thus pressure (force per unit area or newtons per square metre) can also be quoted in bars (1 bar = 10^5 N m^{-2}), and volume can be quoted in litres. Similarly, until such time as a new name may be adopted for the kilogramme as the basic unit of mass, the gramme will often be used both as a basic unit (i.e. to avoid the absurd symbol mkg) and also in association with numerical prefixes (e.g. μg).

Undoubtedly, the introduction of such a system will take time, and the old units will persist alongside the new. Indeed, in some fields it is possible that the new units will never be accepted. A glance at Table 2.6 will reveal immediately that there are a number of awkward conversions to be made. However, there is

TABLE 2.6. Examples of old units with S.I. equivalents.

Physical quantity	Unit	Equivalent
Length	ångstrom	10^{-10} m, i.e. 0·1 nm or 100 pm
	inch	0·0254 m
	foot	0·3048 m
	yard	0·9144 m
	mile	1·60934 km
Area	square inch	645·16 mm^2
	square foot	0·092903 m^2
	square yard	0·836127 m^2
	square mile	2·58999 km^2
Volume	cubic inch	$1·63871 \times 10^{-5}$ m^3
	cubic foot	0·0283168 m^3
	U.K. gallon	0·004546092 m^3
Mass	Pound	0·45359237 kg
Density	pound/cubic inch	$2·76799 \times 10^4$ kg m^{-3}
	pound/cubic foot	16·0185 kg m^{-3}
Force	dyne	10^{-5} N
	poundal	0·138255 N
	pound-force	4·44822 N
	kilogramme-force	9·80665 N
Pressure	atmosphere	101·325 kN m^{-2}
	torr	133·322 N m^{-2}
	pound (f)/sq. in.	6894·76 N m^{-2}
Energy	erg	10^{-7} J
	calorie (I.T.)	4·1868 J
	B.t.u.	1055·06 J
	foot pound (f)	1·35582 J
Power	horse power	745·700 W
Temperature	degree Fahrenheit	$t/°\text{F} = \frac{9}{5}T/°\text{C} + 32$

no doubt that the introduction of S.I. units will do much to improve international communication.

FURTHER READING

Metrication in Scientific Journals. The Royal Society Conference of Editors (1968). The Royal Society, London.

Scientific Tables. Documenta Geigy (1968) 7th ed. J. R. Geigy, S.A., Basle.

HILL D.W. (1969) The application of SI Units to anaesthesia. *British Journal of Anaesthesia*, **41**, 1053.

SOCRATES G. & SAPPER L.J. (1969) *SI and Metrication Conversion Tables.* Newnes-Butterworth, London.

3

Electricity and Electronics

A great deal of measuring apparatus employs electronics in some form or other. Fortunately, it is rarely necessary for the user of a piece of apparatus to have a detailed knowledge of electronics. It is, however, much easier to comprehend the principles on which the instruments are based if one has at least an understanding of basic electronic terminology. This chapter is not intended to be a full exposition of medical electronics, but aims to provide a glossary of terms used later in the book, and to assist those with no previous knowledge to form a mental picture of the subject. Some readers may find it convenient to pass over this chapter and refer back to it if necessary. A more detailed coverage can be found in a variety of textbooks. Whitfield (1959) is extremely useful for beginners. Cornsweet (1963) provides a good introduction to some do-it-yourself circuit designing, and a comprehensive coverage of the electronics involved in medical apparatus is given by Hill (1965).

Direct current

Ohm's Law and resistance. When an electrical potential difference E (sometimes called an electromotive force, or e.m.f.) is applied across a resistor R, the current I which flows (Fig. 3.1) depends on the resistance offered by the resistor. Ohm's Law states the relationship between these quantities as:

$$I = \frac{E}{R}$$

from which it can be seen that if R is large, a smaller current flows for any given potential difference. The resistor hinders the flow of current, and this resistance has the same value whatever the current or potential difference. The current measured is

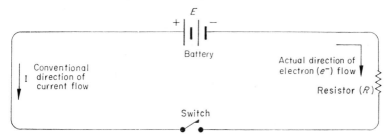

FIG. 3.1. A simple circuit illustrating Ohm's Law.

actually a flow of electrons travelling from negative to positive terminals.

Alternating current

Capacitance. If two conductors are separated by an insulator, the resulting *capacitor* has the property of storing electrons when a potential difference is applied to its terminals. The electrons can be thought of as being squeezed together on the negative plate, until their mutual repulsion is equal and opposite to the applied potential. The excess of electrons on this plate exerts an electrostatic force to drive electrons off the other plate. The unit of capacitance is the *farad*, which is the capacity to store 1 coulomb of charge for an applied potential difference of 1 volt.

If a capacitor is inserted into a direct current circuit, as in Fig. 3.2, and the switch is turned to position B, there will be an initial flow of electrons, which will quickly fall to zero. As there is no electrical continuity across the capacitor, the circuit

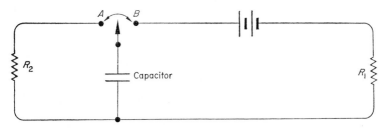

FIG. 3.2. Capacitor and resistors in a simple d.c. circuit.

is incomplete: it is still an *open circuit*, and the capacitor offers an infinite resistance to a direct current. The behaviour of the circuit immediately after the switch is changed to position A or B, however, is rather different, for electrons must flow to build up the charge on the capacitor and they will flow in the opposite direction when the capacitor is discharged. This is analogous to what happens when an alternating source of e.m.f. is applied, and providing the capacitor has not built up an appreciable

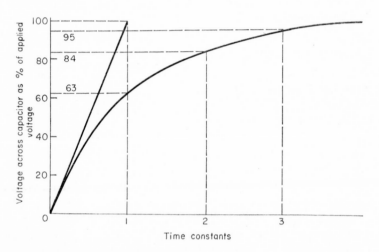

FIG. 3.3. Pattern of charging of a capacitor. Voltage is the voltage developed across a capacitor as a percentage of the applied voltage. Time is expressed in time constants.

back-e.m.f. due to its stored charge before the current reverses, the capacitor appears to conduct freely. Of course, no electrons are actually passing across the capacitor, but for every electron that flows onto one plate, another leaves the opposite plate. In an alternating current circuit, therefore, capacitors conduct electricity. At the moment following reversal of the e.m.f., the current flowing into the capacitor is maximal, but thereafter the electrons stored on the capacitor plate exert a gradually increasing back-potential which reduces the current. At all instances the rate of change of this back-potential is proportional to the back-potential already existing: this is tantamount to saying that the capacitor charges in an exponential fashion (Waters & Mapleson 1964). This is illustrated in Fig. 3.3. Such an exponential process must have a *time constant*. The time constant is the length of time that 100 per cent change would take if the initial rate of change were maintained. It can be shown that 63 per cent of the final value is reached in one time constant; in another time constant 63 per cent of the remaining difference is reached, i.e., 63 per cent + (63/100 × 37 per cent) = 84 per cent. In three time constants, 84 + (63/100 × 16) = 95 per cent of the total change will have occurred, and so on. A large capacitor holds more electrons than a small one and will take longer to charge or discharge; similarly, the rate of charge or discharge will be slower through a high resistor than through a low one, since there will be a smaller flow of current at every potential difference. It is obvious, therefore, that the time constant of any capacitance–resistance combination depends on both capacitance and resistance. In fact, the time constant T (in seconds) is the product of the capacitance in *farads*, multiplied by the resistance in *ohms*:

$$T = RC$$

Inductance. When a current flows through a conductor it induces a magnetic field around the conductor, the strength of the field being proportional to the current. As soon as the current is switched on the magnetic field builds up. During this process the field moves out at right-angles to the wire. If the wire is wound into a coil, the lines of force cut the wire and induce an e.m.f. in it which is opposite in direction to the flow of current, the induced e.m.f. being proportional to the rate of change of the current. When the circuit is 'made' the rate of change of current is maximal, and therefore the induced back-e.m.f. is maximal. As the rate of change of current decreases, so does the back-e.m.f. The back-e.m.f. thus limits the rate of rise of current, which consequently attains its full value in an exponential fashion. When the current is switched off the collapsing field induces an e.m.f., which tends to keep the current flowing. This induced voltage appears across the switch contacts and often results in a spark discharge. Inductance, then, introduces a kind of electrical inertia into the system and the current in the circuit lags behind the applied e.m.f.

Phase-shift in a.c. circuits

It is customary to analyse the behaviour of a.c. circuits by reference to their handling of a simple sine wave. Such a wave is illustrated on the right-hand side of Fig. 3.4. Now a sine wave can be thought of as a linear projection of the point 'O' moving with uniform velocity around the circle ABCD. The wavelength,

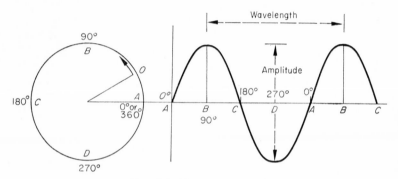

Fig. 3.4. Simple sine wave.

which is the distance between two successive peaks or troughs, can therefore be given the dimensions of angular measurement and thought of as 360°. The distance from A to B, B to C, etc., each of which can be seen to be one-quarter of a complete cycle, can likewise be spoken of as being 90°. An identical second wave which was just passing through zero when the first wave has reached a peak would be one quarter of a cycle, or 90° *out of phase*. This is illustrated in Fig. 3.5. If a wave is delayed, it is likewise described as experiencing a *phase shift*, and the duration of the delay, although strictly a measurement in time, is often more conveniently measured in degrees and spoken of as the *phase angle*. It is important to realize that if two sine waves of different frequencies are both delayed by a similar absolute amount of time, they are delayed by different phase angles. As electronic circuits treat complex waves as though they were mixtures of sine waves, such an occurrence would change the shape of the complex wave, a process known as phase distortion. Inductances and capacitances both introduce a phase difference between the voltage applied to the circuit and the current that actually flows. In the case of an inductance, the inductance acts as an inertia, and the current that flows is always lagging behind the voltage that is being applied, the delay always

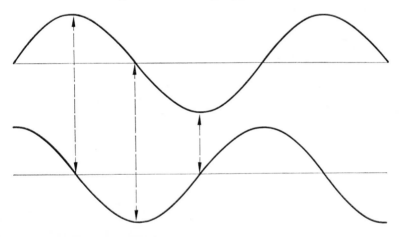

Fig. 3.5. Sine waves of identical frequency, 90° out of phase, the lower one being 90° ahead of the upper.

amounting to 90°. In the case of the capacitor, the voltage across the capacitor cannot be developed until a flow of current has put the charge on the plates, and so the voltage developed across the capacitor always lags behind the current flowing in the circuit, and again the difference between the voltage and the current is 90°.

Reactance. A resistance always has the same ohmic value, whether the current is constant or changing. Inductances and capacitances, however, behave quite differently in a.c. circuits and d.c. circuits. At normal temperatures inductances have a constant inherent ohmic resistance to a steady current, but

oppose any change of current. Since the opposition is proportional to the *rate of change* of the current, the apparent resistance
of an inductance increases as the frequency increases. This
opposition to current flow in an inductance is termed reactance,
and is analogous to resistance in d.c. circuits; it is, therefore,
also measured in ohms. It is linearly dependent on both inductance and frequency according to the formula:

$$\text{reactance } (X_L) \text{ in ohms} = 2\pi.f.L \qquad \text{(see Fig. 3.6)}$$

where $f =$ frequency (Hz)

$L =$ inductance in henrys (H)

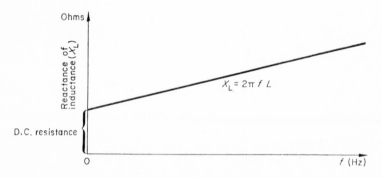

Fig. 3.6. Reactance of an inductance with frequency.

A capacitance has an infinite resistance to a direct current,
but passes an alternating current. In this case, the faster the
current reverses, the less charge builds up on the plates and the
lower the back-e.m.f. A capacitor, therefore, offers progressively
less resistance, the higher the frequency, according to the
formula:

$$\text{reactance } (X_C) \text{ in ohms} = \frac{1}{2\pi.f.C} \qquad \text{(see Fig. 3.7)}$$

where $C =$ capacitance in farads (F)

$f =$ frequency (Hz)

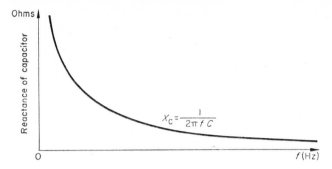

Fig. 3.7. Reactance of a capacitance with frequency.

Impedance

There are thus three sources of opposition to current flow in circuits to which alternating voltages are applied: resistance, inductive reactance, and capacitative reactance. It is often of importance to know the combined effect of these, the resultant at any frequency being known as the *impedance* of the circuit at that frequency. To arrive at the value of the impedance, which is in ohms, the various values cannot be added directly because of the phase differences between voltage and current. Since inductance and capacitance have directly opposite phase effects, they tend to cancel each other out, and their combined reactance is arrived at by subtracting capacitative reactance from inductive reactance. To combine this resultant reactance with resistance, however, account has to be taken of the fact that they are 90° out of phase. The solution may be achieved graphically using vectors whose lengths represent the resistance and the reactance (Fig. 3.8). The resultant (Z) then represents the impedance of the circuit. Those who recall Pythagoras' theorem concerning the lengths of the sides of a right-angled triangle will see that this can be expressed by the formula:

$$Z = \sqrt{\{R^2 + (X_L - X_C)^2\}}$$

where R = resistance
X_L = reactance due to impedance
X_C = reactance due to capacitance.

The above is true when the elements are in series. If the elements are in parallel, a more complicated situation arises, but this is not relevant to this book.

Note that when a circuit contains both reactance and resistance, the current and voltage must necessarily be out of phase. The angle θ in Fig. 3.8 represents the phase angle between the current and voltage in such a circuit. Since reactance is frequency dependent, phase shift will also vary with frequency.

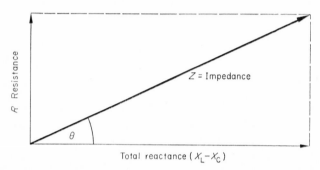

Fig. 3.8. Graphical method of determining impedance (Z) and phase difference (θ).

Resonance

Since the impedance of a capacitor decreases whilst the impedance of an inductance increases as the frequency increases, there is always a frequency at which these impedances are equal. Because of the phase difference they then cancel each other, and at that frequency the impedance is purely resistive and at a minimum value. This is known as the *resonant frequency* of the circuit. By incorporating a variable capacitor or inductance in the circuit it can be tuned to a particular frequency. If these two circuit elements are placed in parallel, the reverse occurs, and the circuit then offers an infinitely high resistance at the resonant frequency.

AMPLIFIERS

The limit to the degree of amplification which can be achieved by an amplifier is set by the signal/noise ratio. Methods for the elimination of source noise were discussed in Chapter 1. However, noise also arises in the amplifier and, although it can be reduced by proper design and construction, it can never be completely eliminated.

For perfect reproduction of an input signal all the frequencies contained in the signal should be equally amplified. Unfortunately this degree of perfection is never achieved and there is always a range of frequencies within which the degree of amplification is reasonably constant, but outside which there is a relative attenuation of the output signal. The acceptable *bandwidth* of an amplifier is usually taken to be the range of frequencies throughout which there is less than 50 per cent relative loss. If the power or voltage gain at any frequency is less than half as great as the optimum achieved by the amplifier, the frequency is said to be outside the band-width of the amplifier.

Because human sensory systems tend to appreciate logarithmic changes in stimulus as linear changes in sensation (e.g. a light emitting ten times as much power seems twice as bright) changes in power or relative differences in power are often measured on a logarithmic scale.

The primary unit of change of power on this scale is the *bel*. The bel is the logarithm of the relative differences between two powers. A 10-fold change in power is therefore 1 bel ($\log 10 = 1\cdot0$). A 100-fold change is likewise 2 bels ($\log 100 = 2\cdot0$). A subdivision of this unit is the *decibel* (dB), 10 dB being equal to 1 bel. The acceptable band-width of an amplifier is usually taken to be the range of frequencies which are amplified with less than a 3 dB loss. Because of the logarithmic nature of the scale this is much more than it looks, and amounts to a reduction of 50 per cent:

$$\frac{\text{maximum output power}}{\text{power of attenuated frequencies}} = \frac{2}{1}$$

$$\log 2 = 0\cdot301 \text{ bel} \qquad 10 \times 0\cdot301 = 3\cdot01 \text{ dB}$$

Similarly, a 30 dB change in power is a 1000-fold change, i.e. 500 times as great as 3 dB.

In amplifiers the input signal voltage controls the flow of
2*

current between the anode and cathode of a valve, or between the emitter and collector of a transistor. The degree of amplification which can be produced is limited to a factor of two or three hundred. To amplify the signal further it is necessary to introduce extra stages. If one stage amplifies 50 times, then the gain of two stages will be $50 \times 50 = 2500$, and so on. Each of these stages must be coupled to the next and it is the method of coupling which gives rise to the terms *a.c.* and *d.c. amplifiers*. If the signals to be amplified have a frequency of more than 1 Hz (i.e. the signal is a.c.) *capacitance* or, rarely, *transformer*, *coupling* may be used. However, if the signal fluctuates at a rate of less than 1 Hz or is relatively steady it is necessary to employ *direct coupling*. Unfortunately, in direct-coupled amplifiers slow changes in the amplifier characteristics or power supplies cause changes in the output which are indistinguishable from a signal. Great care is therefore taken to minimise baseline drift in such amplifiers. Gain stability is usually ensured by employing the principle of *negative feedback*, in which a proportion of the output voltage is fed back to the input. It is arranged that this feedback is 180° out of phase with the input so that it decreases the overall gain of the amplifier but improves the gain stability.

Although the design of d.c. amplifiers has greatly improved over the past decade, there is still a place for techniques which enable signals having a d.c. component to be handled by an a.c. amplifier. One method is to convert the signal to an alternating one, to amplify that signal and then to *rectify* it to obtain the amplified d.c. signal. A common method of achieving this is to inject an alternating *carrier wave* which can be modified (or *modulated*) by the signal, by varying either its amplitude or its frequency in a way which is characteristic of the signal. The modulated wave is then amplified or otherwise processed, and finally demodulated to produce the amplified biological variable.

Another method of converting biological direct currents into convenient alternating currents is to chop up the signal into small intervals which are all interspersed with a return to zero current. This signal is now amplified as an alternating signal and then 'smoothed out'. The possible frequency response with such *chopper amplifiers* depends on the chopper frequency and the time constants of the smoothing circuit, and is considerably less than can be obtained with carrier-wave amplifiers.

Modern developments have made it possible to construct extremely stable and compact d.c. amplifiers which, by suitable coupling, can be made to perform various arithmetic operations such as summation, integration, differentiation and multiplication. They are therefore described as zero-frequency or operational amplifiers and form the basic units in analogue computers (Chapter 5). They are fully described by Hill (1967).

Differentiation and integration
It is difficult to explain these terms accurately without reference to calculus, but for present purposes a few examples must suffice.

Differentiation is a mathematical process which yields the rate of change of a variable with respect to another variable, usually time. For example, the differential of distance travelled is velocity, since

$$\text{velocity} = \frac{\text{distance}}{\text{time}}$$

Similarly, the rate of change of velocity is acceleration and acceleration is therefore the differential of velocity. Another example of the use of differentiation is provided by one of the techniques used to assess cardiac contractility. The rise in intraventricular pressure during isometric contraction is recorded and the rate of rise is obtained by differentiating the pressure signal.

Integration is the opposite of differentiation, and can best be illustrated by reference to Fig. 3.9. If gas flows at a rate of 5 litres per minute for 5 minutes, a volume of 25 litres must have passed through the flowmeter. This answer was achieved by multiplying the flow rate by the duration of flow, but could equally well have been obtained by adding the volume of gas passed each minute or second or by measuring the area under the graph. In this case volume is the integral of flow rate with respect to time, and the process of adding each of the volumes resulting from a known gas flow passing for a given time is termed

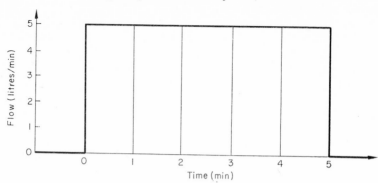

FIG. 3.9. Graph illustrating flow plotted against time.

integration. Suppose now that the gas flow was not constant and followed the pattern shown in Fig. 3.10. In order to determine the volume it would be necessary to divide the area under the graph into a series of narrow rectangles and then add the volumes represented by these rectangles. The narrower these rectangles were drawn the greater would be the accuracy with which volume could be calculated. Volume could also be calculated by measuring the area under the curve by planimetry or by cutting out the curve and weighing the paper. By the use of suitable circuits this process of integration can be carried out electronically. The commonest examples are the integration of the signal generated

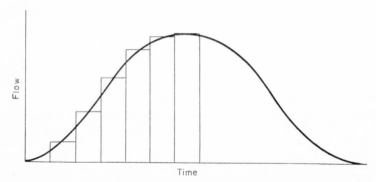

FIG. 3.10. Record of inspiratory flow rate.

by the pressure difference across a pneumotachograph (page 125) to yield a signal proportional to volume, or the integration of the areas under cardiac output or gas chromatograph curves. Integration is also used to determine the mean value of a rapidly changing signal, such as a blood-pressure trace.

The black box

An important concept is to regard a group of electronic circuits as a 'black box' which has input terminals and output terminals. When an electronic signal is fed to the input terminals, the source of the signal 'sees' the box as offering a certain impedance. If the impedance of the box is high it will take minimal current from the source, and it will therefore not matter if the source has itself a high impedance. On the other hand, if the black box takes a lot of current, the source 'sees' this as a low impedance. In recording biological signals, such a loading of the source is undesirable, for if the source has a high impedance, this will greatly reduce the current available to the box, and so will modify the signal recorded. In a similar fashion the output impedance of the black box is seen by the next 'box', usually a recording instrument. It can be shown that the maximum power transfer between two 'black boxes' occurs when their respective input and output impedances are the same. Matching of input and output impedances is therefore of great importance.

Wheatstone bridge

This configuration is extremely common as a measuring arrangement. Its simplest form is shown in Fig. 3.11. G is a sensitive current detector. When no current is detected, the points A and B must be at the same potential. This condition occurs when the ratio of the resistance of P to Q is the same as the ratio of S to the unknown resistance R. It is equally true that the ratio of P to S is the same as the ratio of Q to R. Using known resistances in S, it is possible to measure an unknown, R. More commonly, the circuit is used as a null detector, and an arbitrary number on an accurately scaled variable resistor at S will then be proportional to any change in R. This principle is used for measuring the change of resistance of strain-gauge elements in blood-pressure transducers (p. 93). Note that it is possible to double the sensitivity by incorporating two such elements in appropriate arms of the bridge. If they are both increasing or decreasing in resistance together, they should be placed in opposite arms, e.g., P and R in Fig. 3.11. If, however, the elements are so arranged that one element is stretched while the other is compressed, and consequently the resistance in one is increasing while that in the other is decreasing, then sensitivity is increased by

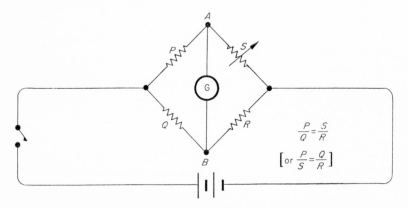

FIG. 3.11. A Wheatstone bridge circuit. When A and B are equipotential $P/Q = S/R$, or $P/S = Q/R$.

placing them in adjacent arms, such as P and Q. The Wheatstone bridge can also be used whenever some detected quantity is linearly (or at least predictably) related to a change of resistance, by calibrating the meter in terms of the change of resistance. If an alternating voltage is used to energise the bridge, both capacitances and inductances can be incorporated as resistance elements. The detector is then usually an a.c. valve voltmeter instead of a galvanometer.

Certain other electronic topics appear elsewhere in the text; they include the cathode-ray oscilloscope (Chapter 4), photomultiplier tubes (Chapter 6), and biological amplifiers (Chapter 14).

REFERENCES

CORNSWEET T.N. (1963) *The Design of Electric Circuits in the Behavioural Sciences*. John Wiley & Sons, Inc., New York and London.

HILL D.W. (1965) *Principles of Electronics in Medical Research*. Butterworth, London.

HILL D.W. (1968) *Physics Applied to Anaesthesia*. Butterworth, London.

WHITFIELD I.C. (1959) *An Introduction to Electronics for Physiological Workers*. 2nd ed. Macmillan, London.

Waters D.J. & Mapleson W.W. (1964) Exponentials and the anaesthetist. *Anaesthesia*, **19**, 274.

4

Recorders

Recording and display are usually carried out by two separate instruments. However, in some systems the signals can be easily visualised on the paper while the recording is being made, thereby eliminating the need for display, whilst in others the display itself is photographed for record purposes.

Recorders may be divided into three main types: direct writers, in which a writing arm makes a direct imprint on the paper; photographic, in which the impression is made by a beam of light; and magnetic, in which the data is stored on magnetic tape or in a computer 'store'. Before describing recorders in more detail, certain factors which affect their performance must be mentioned.

Frequency response
The frequency response of recorders in which there is a movable writing arm is determined by the undamped natural frequency and the degree of damping (see Chapter 8). The relationship between these two also determines the degree of phase shift.

In most recorders the writing arm is activated by a current passing through a small coil which is suspended in a powerful magnetic field. The degree of rotation of the coil, and hence the excursion of the writing arm, is proportional to the current flowing through it. This mechanism is known as a moving-coil galvanometer. The other system commonly used for driving the writing arm is the moving-iron system, in which a permanent magnet (attached to the writing arm) is mounted inside a fixed coil. A variation in signal strength in the fixed coil varies the strength of the electromagnetic field and so alters the position of the permanent magnet and writing arm. In either case it is the inertia of the driving system plus writing arm which limits the frequency response of the recorder. Normally the response of a recorder is 'flat' (i.e. response is proportional to input), up to about two-thirds of the resonant frequency of the system, providing that the system is critically damped (see Chapter 8). Above this frequency distortion occurs. To obtain the maximum frequency response from a recorder it is therefore necessary to make the resonant frequency as high as possible. This is accomplished by reducing the mass of the moving parts of the system.

The writing arm with the least mass is a beam of electrons. This principle is used in the cathode-ray oscilloscope, and it is this instrument which is preferred when an extremely high frequency response is required. Moving-coil or moving-iron galvanometers have a very much lower frequency response, the maximum being about 8000 cycles per second (8 kHz). To maintain this high frequency response it is necessary to minimise the mass of the coil and writing arm. The easiest way of doing this is to attach a small mirror to the coil. The rotation of the coil is then detected by reflecting a beam of light onto the recording paper. This unit is known as a mirror galvanometer. Unfortunately, if the coil is small, sensitivity is reduced : sensitivity can be increased by lengthening the light path by reflecting the light beam back and forth between fixed mirrors before it impinges on the recording paper, or by increasing the density of the magnetic field surrounding the coil.

Another instrument based on the moving-coil galvanometer is the ink-jet recorder. In this unit a small jet is attached to the coil. Ink is forced out of the jet under pressure and impinges on the paper. The frequency response is somewhat reduced in this instrument—about 500 Hz maximum—but the running costs are low, since no photographic emulsion is required. In later versions of this recorder the jet is attached to a small permanent magnet suspended in an electromagnetic field which varies with signal strength. This is linear up to about 700 Hz.

The addition of a pen to the driving unit results in a very great reduction in frequency response, most pen recorders having a flat response up to a maximum of 75–100 Hz. Potentiometric

recorders have the lowest speed of response of all, some taking
up to 2 seconds to achieve full scale deflection.

Linearity

It is important that the amplitude of the displacement should
be linearly related to the amplitude of the input signal. In

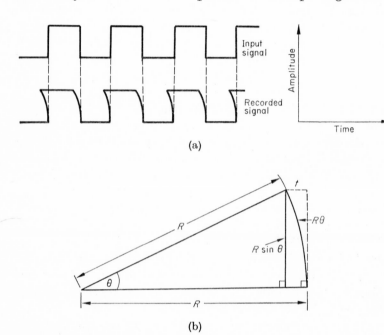

(a)

(b)

FIG. 4.1. (a) Record of square wave deflection showing curvilinear
coordinates of pen recorder. (b) Sine distortion. R represents the
length of the writing arm. 't' = time error.

recorders employing a lever or optical writing arm there are two
sources of distortion which tend to produce alinearity.

Sine distortion. Since a pen recorder writes in an arc, its vertical
coordinates are curvilinear. (Fig. 4.1a). If the angular displacement is θ the vertical displacement of the recorded signal is
$R\sin\theta$, where R is the length of the writing arm. The length of
the arc is, however, $R\theta$, where θ is in radians. For deflections

up to about 15° the error of the recorded displacement of the pen tip is smaller than the error introduced by the thickness of the ink trace (0·5 mm). Of more importance is the fact that sine distortion introduces a timing error (Fig. 4.1b). Although this can be overcome by the use of curvilinear coordinates on the paper, this stratagem often proves unsatisfactory, since the shape of the waveform may be grossly distorted.

Sine distortion may be overcome by mounting the writing arm vertically so that it writes on paper which is pulled along a curved

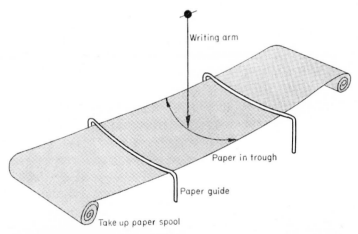

Fig. 4.2. The use of a curved trough and vertical writing arm to overcome sine distortion.

trough (Fig. 4.2). It is, however, difficult to apply this technique when multi-channel recording is being employed. A more satisfactory alternative is to draw the paper over a knife-edge and to use a heated stylus to mark heat-sensitive paper.* The heated stylus is usually about 1–2 cm long and is mounted at the tip of the writing arm in its long axis. The knife-edge is mounted at right-angles to the direction of travel of the paper. When the writing arm is deflected laterally the point of contact of the

---

* This type of paper has a black base and is covered with a thin layer of white cellulose. When the cellulose is melted the black base shows through.

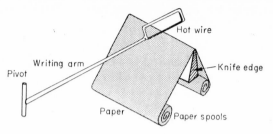

FIG. 4.3. The use of a heated stylus and knife-edge to overcome sine distortion.

heated stylus with the knife-edge moves towards the tip of the writing arm. This, in effect, lengthens the arm as it moves laterally and so ensures that the time coordinate is unaffected by lateral displacement of the writing arm (Fig. 4.3). In a few recorders sine distortion is overcome by lengthening the arm mechanically. To accomplish this without decreasing frequency response requires engineering of high precision: such recorders are therefore very expensive (Fig. 4.4).

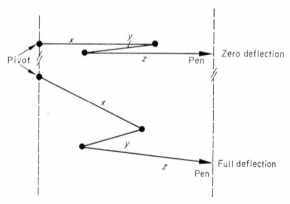

FIG. 4.4. The use of a mechanical linkage to lengthen the writing arm and so obviate sine distortion.

Tangent distortion. Whilst the use of a heated stylus and knife-edge ensures that the time coordinates of multi-channel recordings are correctly aligned it introduces another source of error, namely, tangent distortion (Fig. 4.5). Whilst the true deflection is the arc $= R\theta$ the measured displacement along the vertical coordinate is $R\tan\theta$. This form of distortion can lead to quite a large degree of alinearity, particularly when large angular displacements occur as in ink jet and photographic recorders. It can, however, be corrected electronically.

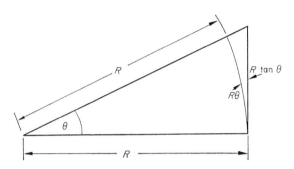

FIG. 4.5. Tangent distortion. R represents the length of the writing arm. $R\tan\theta$ indicates the deflection recorded by the heated stylus.

TYPES OF RECORDER

Direct writers

The disadvantages of pen recorders have already been outlined. Nevertheless their relative simplicity, the immediacy of the image and the cheapness of the recording paper make them a popular choice for many types of recording (e.g. E.E.G., E.C.G.) where linearity and sine distortion are not important. By suitable modification many of the disadvantages can be minimised. Heat-sensitive paper is much more expensive than ordinary recording paper, but the use of a heated stylus is one of the easiest ways of overcoming sine distortion. Other methods of producing an image are a cold stylus writing on pressure-sensitive paper and the use of 'Teledeltos' paper. The latter conducts electricity and an imprint is produced where a current flows from the pen onto the paper.

All direct recorders display *hysteresis*, i.e. the pen does not return exactly to zero after it has been deflected by the current. By correct design of the spring which returns the pen to zero, hysteresis can be reduced to less than 2 per cent of the maximum deflection.

The flat frequency response of most pen recorders is limited to 75–100 Hz. A typical sensitivity is 1 mA or 100 μA for full-scale deflection.

Photographic recorders

Cathode-ray oscilloscope. When this instrument is used for display the trace can be photographed directly with a time exposure. It is often difficult to adjust the trace to the correct brightness at the first attempt, but the use of a Polaroid-Land camera enables a print to be obtained immediately so that the appropriate adjustments may be made.

By holding the shutter open for prolonged periods and triggering the time base from a fixed point on a repetitive signal, photographic averaging can be accomplished. The signal trace passes over the same points on the photographic emulsion at each sweep and so exposes this part of the film maximally, whilst the random variations in the trace due to noise are spread over a wide area of emulsion, where they produce a generalised haziness. By adjusting the brightness of the oscilloscope trace and the sensitivity of the film, it is thus possible to achieve a clear image of the trace, free from noise artefacts.

When prolonged periods of recording are required the time base on the oscilloscope may be switched off and the film moved continuously through the camera. The oscillations of the light spots in the Y-axis then produce continuous traces on the film. This form of recording greatly enhances the versatility of the instrument but some care is necessary to ensure correct exposure.

Although the oscilloscope gun itself requires a fairly high voltage to produce a deflection (e.g. 10 volts/cm deflection) high gain amplifiers are usually incorporated in the chassis so that input signals as small as 100 μV can produce a 1 cm deflection. Although a certain amount of experience with the technique is necessary to produce good records, there is no alternative when one wishes to record components of a waveform having a frequency greater than about 5 kHz.

Mirror galvanometers. Photographic recorders utilising the mirror galvanometer (Fig. 1.4) have been used for many years, but they have suffered from the disadvantage that the trace had to be developed and fixed before the image could be inspected. However, the introduction of ultra-violet light sensitive paper, on which an image appears after a delay of about 15 seconds, has once again brought the mirror galvanometer recorder back into popularity. The image on this paper is semi-permanent, but the paper blackens if it is exposed for prolonged periods to bright light. The image can be preserved by chemical treatment or by spraying the paper with a protective yellow varnish.

Galvanometer recorders have a number of advantages. Many channels (sometimes up to 50 or 100) can be recorded on the same strip of paper and the traces can be overlapped so that each trace can sweep the full width of the paper. Identification marks can be superimposed on each trace and a time scale and calibration grid can be printed onto the paper as it passes through the recorder. The light spots can also be projected onto a ground-glass screen so that the zero and calibration points can be adjusted and the recording monitored visually. Perhaps the greatest advantage is the wide choice of galvanometers, which enables the galvanometer to be matched exactly to the character of the input signal. Since each galvanometer is carried as a complete unit in a cylinder about 6 cm × 0·5 cm, it is a simple matter to change galvanometers when required.

Choice of a galvanometer

The sensitivity of a galvanometer depends on the length of the optical writing arm (mirror to paper distance) and on the deflection of the mirror produced by a given current or voltage. The deflection can be increased by increasing the density of the magnetic field or by increasing the size of the coil. There is a limit to the density of the magnetic field which can be achieved and the larger the coil the lower is the undamped natural frequency. Although the sensitivity is also affected by the internal resistance of the galvanometer, it is approximately inversely proportional to the square of the natural frequency.

There is therefore no advantage to be gained from using a galvanometer with a higher frequency response than that required for the purpose in hand. For this reason the first step in choosing a galvanometer is to decide on the maximum frequency which it will be called upon to handle. The undamped natural frequency is then calculated by multiplying this by a factor of 1·6 since, if it is correctly damped, the frequency response should be flat to 60–65 per cent of its natural frequency.

In addition to frequency response and sensitivity it is necessary to consider the relative importance of three other characteristics namely, damping, phase-shift and power dissipation. It is pointed out in Chapter 8 that correct damping is essential if the galvanometer is to reproduce a signal accurately. It has been found by experience that the optimal value of damping for the maximum flat frequency range is 64·5 per cent of critical: this gives the best practical compromise between overshoot and frequency response and under ideal conditions it is possible to achieve a flat response (±2 per cent) up to 67 per cent of the galvanometer's natural frequency. This degree of damping results in about a 7 per cent overshoot in response to a square wave signal (Fig. 8.20).

The phase angle (i.e. the change of phase between input and recorded signal) is determined by the natural frequency of the galvanometer and the damping ratio. When damping is about 65 per cent of critical there is a fairly linear relationship between phase angle and frequency ratio (ratio of actual frequency to undamped natural frequency of the galvanometer, Fig. 8.21). If it is desired to use galvanometers with different undamped natural frequencies but it is necessary to retain the same phase angle (i.e. delay) for each galvanometer, then the degree of damping must be changed. However, this change in damping will then affect both frequency response and sensitivity.

From these considerations it is apparent that correct damping is of great importance. In galvanometers with undamped natural frequencies up to 300–400 Hz damping is applied electromagnetically, but with galvanometers with undamped natural frequencies above about 1 kHz fluid damping is used. Electromagnetic damping is achieved by inserting a known resistance into the galvanometer circuit so that the reverse current which is induced in the coil by the deflection of the coil produces the required degree of damping. The magnitude of this resistance can only be calculated if the resistance of the source of current is known, for optimal conditions exist when the resistance of the source equals the resistance of the damping resistance. When these resistances are not equal, a series, or parallel resistance, may need to be incorporated in the circuit. Details are given in the manufacturers' literature.

Some typical values for galvanometer characteristics are given in Table 4.1.

TABLE 4.1.

Natural frequency (Hz)	Flat frequency response (±5 per cent) (Hz)	Galvanometer sensitivity	
		(mA/cm)	(mV/cm)
35	20	0·0008	0·038
450	300	0·05	6·0
1000	600	0·34	25
5000	3000	25	1050

Potentiometric

This type of recorder is used when it is desired to inscribe a curve over a wide strip of recording paper (e.g. 15–25 cm) with high accuracy. Sensitivity can be made very high (range 1–100 mV for full-scale deflection) but the response is slow, the pen sometimes taking up to 2 seconds to traverse the full width of the paper.

The recorder is based on the standard potentiometric circuit, which is used for measuring an electromotive force (e.m.f., see Chapter 3). When the e.m.f. developed across the resistance of the slide wire is out of balance with the e.m.f. being measured, a current flows. In the potentiometer this current is displayed

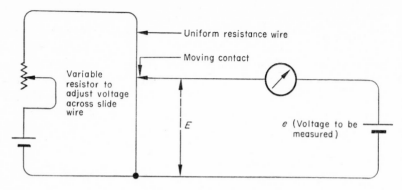

Fig. 4.6. Principle of potentiometric recorder.

on a meter (Fig. 4.6). In the potentiometric recorder the current is amplified and used to drive a motor which adjusts the contact on the slide wire until the two e.m.f.'s balance. The chart pen is attached to the sliding contact and therefore follows the input e.m.f. (Fig. 4.7).

At the point of balance a potentiometer recorder draws no current from the signal source. Its input resistance is then high. However, when the recorder is off balance a current is drawn from the source and the resistance of the recorder and the resistance of the source then become important. If for example

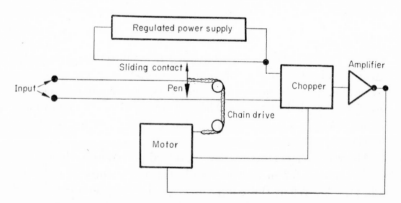

Fig. 4.7. Diagram to illustrate mechanism of potentiometric recorder.

the recorder resistance is small and a large current is drawn from a source which has a high resistance, then the response of the recorder may be very sluggish. It is therefore important to match the recorder to the source.

Potentiometric recorders are used in many monitoring applications and for such relatively slow changes as indicator dilution curves or gas chromatograms. Sampling recorders, printing out distinctive marks for a number of different variables in rotation, are used for such applications as the monitoring of temperature from a number of different probes. Another variation is the X-Y recorder, in which two potentiometer movements drive the pen along axes at right-angles to each other. This may be used for plotting two simultaneously altering variables such as pressure/volume loops.

Magnetic tape

This is most useful for temporary storage of data or for prolonged monitoring. It has the additional advantage that a spoken commentary may be recorded on a parallel channel. Usually, tape is used when it is desired to select small periods of a long recording for detailed analysis. These portions of the record can be played back into a direct-writing or photographic recorder at a different speed to obtain a permanent visual record and the tape can then be re-used. Another convenient technique utilises the tape loop. This is a complete loop of tape which can be varied in length to provide a period of recording which suits the chosen application. As the tape passes through the recording head the previous signal is erased and the new signal is recorded. This type of recorder is very useful in patient monitoring. An example is the monitoring of the E.C.G. in patients likely to develop a cardiac arrhythmia or arrest. If the nurse stops the machine when such an arrest occurs the E.C.G. for the previous 5 or 10 minutes will be retained on the tape and can be played back to reveal the pattern of events leading up to the arrest. This type of recorder overcomes the problems imposed by bulky tape spools and enables the recording to be limited to the period most likely to yield useful information.

Ordinary tape recorders are not suitable for most biological work, since much of the input data has a very low frequency component. A frequency or pulse-modulation system must therefore be used.

Another form of magnetic storage is digital storage in a computer. It can be arranged that the waveform is accepted in analogue form and that this waveform is then converted to a digital form by sampling at frequent intervals. These digits can then be preserved in the magnetic store in a computer. This form of storage facilitates subsequent manipulation of the data. However, the method requires a large store and is very expensive. The applications are, accordingly, rather restricted at the present time.

5

Computers

There are two types of computers, analogue and digital, but both have the ability to carry out mathematical processes at a rate which far exceeds that of the brain or, indeed, of any standard desk calculator. Although the calculations are performed in a similar manner in both the desk calculator and computer, it is the use of electronic circuitry in the latter which is responsible for the enormous increase in speed.

The difference between the two types of computer is probably best illustrated by a simple example such as the addition of two numbers. In the digital computer these two numbers are stored in the form of a number of coded electrical impulses in a magnetic store. When the addition is performed these impulses are added and the result is then decoded back into figures. When this sum is performed by an analogue computer each figure is represented by a voltage and the two voltages are then added by an electronic circuit. The output voltage then represents the sum of these two figures and can be read from a meter or graphical display.

ANALOGUE COMPUTERS

By definition an analogue computer is a machine which uses a physical quantity to represent each variable in the problem being solved, the magnitude of the physical quantity being made proportional to the magnitude of the original variable. The analogues most commonly favoured are electrical voltage or mechanical position, but other analogues (e.g. hydraulic models) could also be used. Electrical analogues have many advantages and have now displaced most of the other analogues previously employed. Certain processes, such as integration and differentiation, are particularly suited to solution by analogue computer but many other mathematical processes can also be carried out.

51

A simple example of an analogue computation is shown in Fig. 5.1. The problem is to define how changes in lung compliance and airway resistance will affect the rate of airflow into the lung when a constant pressure is applied to the trachea. In the analogue circuit the pressure is represented by a constant voltage supplied from a battery, the airway resistance is represented by a resistor R and lung compliance is represented by a capacitor C. When the switch S is closed current flows round the circuit and a charge builds up on the capacitor. If the charge on the capacitor is displayed on a meter or oscilloscope it will be seen to rise exponentially. The curve can also be recorded so that the

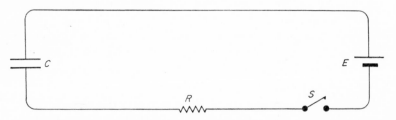

FIG. 5.1. Simple circuit used to simulate the effect of changes in lung compliance and airway resistance on the rate of airflow into the lung. *C* (capacitor) represents lung compliance. *R* (resistor) represents airway resistance. *E* (e.m.f.) represents pressure exerted to drive air into the lung. *S* = switch.

time constant can be calculated. It is now a simple matter to replace the original resistor with one having half the previous value and to repeat the experiment. By varying the resistor and capacitor a whole series of curves can be obtained which illustrate the flow of gas into the lung under different conditions of airway resistance and lung compliance. In this simple example it would have been quite straightforward to calculate the time constant for each set of conditions from the equation

$$T = RC$$

where T = time (in seconds)
R = resistance (in ohms)
C = capacitance (in farads)

However, it can be readily seen that in the case of complex circuits the calculations may become very tedious, whilst the analogue solution may remain very simple. It is in this situation that the analogue computer is of the greatest use.

The foregoing is an example of a *passive* analogue. The components, resistance, and capacitance, behave in a passive way, and the values of voltage and current are the inevitable consequences of the physical conditions. A more sophisticated use of analogue computing methods can be provided by *active* analogues. These use stable d.c. amplifiers, which process the input signal and so render it possible to perform, not only the simple arithmetic functions such as addition and subtraction, but more complex functions such as integration and differentiation. For example, it is now possible to use special-purpose analogue units to integrate a flow measurement to volume, and then to multiply it by a simultaneous measurement of concentration to derive mass per minute.

It will be apparent from this simple description that there are three essential characteristics which must be incorporated into any analogue computer. They are amplitude scaling, time scaling and facilities for programming.

Amplitude scaling. The only quantity which can be measured in the analogue computer is voltage. The first requirement is therefore that the input voltage must be adjusted so that a suitable voltage is available to the machine. This voltage may later be modified in various other parts of the network and it must finally be adjusted so that the output voltage is adequate to drive the selected display unit, whether this be a cathode-ray oscilloscope, meter, or chart recorder. The process of adjusting the voltage at various stages, either by amplification or attenuator units, is known as amplitude scaling.

Time scaling. The time scale of the process analysed on an analogue computer may vary from milliseconds to years. Obviously it is desirable to have a readout time which presents the results in the most compact form (say 30 seconds of recording) and to effect this it is necessary to adjust the time scale so that the ratio of input to output times produces a suitable readout.

Programming. One of the main problems connected with the use of analogue computers is the formulation of the equations necessary to build up the model. Often these must be simplified in order to clarify the result. However, when the machine is programmed it is a very simple matter to change any of the constants used in the equations to allow the effects to be observed.

The programme is usually set up on a patchboard which contains all the input and output sockets of the various circuits contained in the machine. In some computers the patchboard is removable, so that programmes can be set up away from the computer and then attached to it for the period of use. A number of analogue computers suitable for medical use are now available commercially. They are often small enough to sit on a desk-top and are highly versatile.

Analogue computers have been used to investigate theoretically the effect of changing conditions on such matters as the uptake and elimination of anaesthetic agents (Mapleson 1964), the effects of altering ventilation on lung function (Campbell & Brown 1963) and the effect of different patterns of lung inflation on gas exchange during mechanical ventilation (Wald, Murphy & Mazzia 1968). Their use in anaesthetic research has been reviewed by Bellville & Hara (1966). They are a useful teaching aid (Cole *et al.* 1968) and can also guide research work by providing a theoretical analysis which can be validated by experimental observations.

DIGITAL COMPUTERS

This type of computer most commonly receives its input in digital form although analogue-to-digital converters are available and may be used, for example, to convert a graph into a digital input.

Basically, digital computers consist of an input unit, a central processor comprising a store, an arithmetic unit and control unit, and an output unit (Fig. 5.2).

Input unit. This is used to feed instructions and data into the

store. This could be accomplished by the use of a special typewriter on the control unit, but such a method would be slow and
would therefore waste valuable computer time. Most commonly
the data is presented to the input device in the form of holes
punched in paper tape or cards. The holes in the tape or cards
are then 'read' electronically by a tape or card reader, which
transmits the appropriate impulses into the central processor.
Paper tape is punched on a special typewriter which simultaneously prints out a copy of the input data which has been
punched. This provides an essential check. When the tape has
been prepared it is fed into the tape reader. This can usually

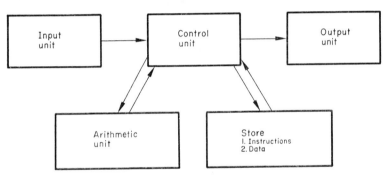

Fig. 5.2. Components of a digital computer.

read 5-, 6-, 7- or 8-channel tape at rates up to 1000 characters
per second. Cards typically contain about 90 characters per card
and a stack of cards can be read at rates up to 600 cards per
minute.

Since the rate at which input data is read is so much greater
than the time taken to punch the tapes, it is customary for there
to be a number of tape or card punches attached to each computer installation. In many cases it is more convenient to have
these machines situated in the departments which are using the
computer, so that data punching can be more easily integrated
with other departmental work.

Central processing unit. This constitutes the main body of the
computer. It consists of a *store* which holds the raw data and

3

the instructions for operating on it, an *arithmetic (or logic) unit* which carries out the actual calculations and a *control unit* which examines the instructions placed in the store and then causes the arithmetic unit to carry out the instructions contained therein.

The store. In an ideal unit the store would have a high capacity and would be capable of immediate access. This, however, would make the cost prohibitive, and most computers therefore utilise a small, fast-access, basic store and a large, slow-access, backing store. The basic store accommodates the instructions and a limited amount of basic data, whilst the backing store is chiefly reserved for storage of large quantities of data which may only be referred to occasionally.

The basic store is usually made up of a large number of ferrite cores situated at the junctions of a lattice of wires. Each ferrite ring can be magnetised in one of two directions, according to the direction of current flow through it. When the store is 'read' the state of magnetism is unaffected and remains in this condition until the core is remagnetised by a new set of data. Each 'location' in the store has a number or 'address' and there may be several hundred thousand addresses in a basic store.

The backing store may be of two types. *A serial backing store* is used to store large quantities of data which may be required serially. It is therefore particularly suited to the storage of patient records which may have to be searched serially for some particular characteristic. Magnetic tape is the medium which is most commonly employed for this purpose, many millions of pieces of information being stored on a single tape. The magnetic tape reader can transfer data to the basic store at rates of up to 30,000 characters per second, but there is, of course, a pronounced delay if the information to be retrieved is at the other end of the tape. To overcome this problem *random access backing stores* are also used. Currently those employed are magnetic drums, discs and cards. These units allow all the data to be located relatively quickly (milliseconds rather than minutes) and the delay is approximately the same wherever the material is situated.

The *arithmetic unit* is very limited in the number of processes which it can carry out, these being strictly similar to a desk calculator (multiply, divide, add, subtract, move decimal point, etc.). The steps in each calculation must therefore be specified in great detail.

The *control unit* is also limited in the number of instructions which it can carry out. The control unit may be addressed by a special typewriter on the console and by the instructions contained in the programme; it is also used to control the input and output units.

The *output unit*. Once again the relative slowness of typing prohibits direct print-out from the computer. The output data is therefore punched out on paper tape (at speeds up to 110 characters per second) and this is subsequently fed into a teleprinter which prints it up at rates of up to 10 characters per second. It is worth noting that even though the output tape is punched at such a high rate it is still necessary for the computer to store its output whilst the punch operates!

Alternative forms of output exist. For example, the output can be displayed graphically on a screen or can be plotted as a series of points on a graph by a digital plotter.

Much development work is at present being undertaken with more direct means of communicating with the computer. With the aid of a 'light pencil', it is possible to enter data directly by writing onto a modified cathode-ray screen. One such system has reached the commercial stage in the application of keeping patients' records. Each ward and laboratory has its own terminal, and can add or retrieve information concerning any patient immediately. By shining the light pencil at an appropriate signal area, the front page of the patient's notes is displayed on the screen. This lists all the contents, such as history, biochemical investigations and temperature chart, and by shining the light pencil at the appropriate heading, the screen display changes to the requested section. If this section contains more information than can be shown on one page, again there is a sub-index page, which titles the wanted section. Further results can be added by teletype associated with the terminal.

This is just one example of an application in which it is convenient to be able to punch and print out data at stations which are remote from the computer. When these remote stations are directly connected to the computer by telephone or direct linkage, the installation is said to be *on line*. To be economically feasible, this has to be associated with *time sharing* resources, which enable the computer to handle a number of different programmes simultaneously. It does this by having sections of memory which hold incoming instructions and data until the machine is free to deal with them. The machine then automatically switches to the next job waiting in the memory. Because of the relative slowness of input and output processes and the fantastically rapid rate at which the central processor can handle material, the delay is hardly, if ever, detectable to the user.

Programming

The problems involved in programming a computer can best be illustrated by a few simple examples.

Suppose the calculation to be performed is $4 \times 6 \times 12$. The first instruction on the programme will read, 'Take the following numbers into the stores shown: store No. 200: 4, store No. 201: 6, store No. 202: 12.' The next instruction will say, 'Begin the calculation: multiply the figure in store 200 by the figure in store 201 and place the answer in store 300.' This will be followed by an instruction: 'Multiply the figure in store 202 by the figure in store 300 and place the answer in store 301. Print out the answer in store 301.' There will finally be an instruction to 'stop'.

It can be seen immediately that the programme must contain detailed instructions about every action to be made by the computer and it must be told when to begin and when to finish.

Such simple programmes are more easily performed on a desk calculator (or even in the head!), but it can be seen that the programme will become extremely complex if many additional steps have to be added. A further example will illustrate another type of problem which occurs.

Suppose the computer has to select from a series of patient

records all patients whose age is greater than 40. The process may then be represented as follows:

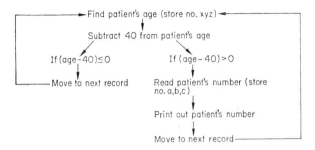

In this case the machine has to make a 'yes' or 'no' decision. If the answer is 'yes' it has to perform one routine, whereas if the answer is 'no' it passes on to the next patient's data in the store and repeats the search. The computer's actions have been summarised in the form of a *flow-diagram* in the example illustrated above and this has then to be translated into detailed instructions on the programme.

Certain actions, such as that illustrated above, occur in many different types of programmes, and it is a waste of time for each individual programmer to have to write out the detailed instructions in full. For this reason manufacturers provide codes which act as a key to common sub-routines. It is then only necessary for the programmer to include this code whenever that particular sub-routine is required. These codes are built up to constitute a language which is matched to the computer being used, the two most common languages in this country being ALGOL and FORTRAN.

From this brief discussion it is evident that the function of a computer depends primarily on the programme. Many months may be required to assemble and test a complex programme, even if it is compiled by a professional programmer, but no matter how simple the programme it is essential to elaborate a flow-diagram first. This is usually the most difficult part of the whole procedure and requires a high degree of critical thought. The flow-diagram may be prepared by the ultimate user or may be prepared by the user in co-operation with a *systems analyst*. After preparation of the flow-diagram the *programmer* translates the processes into a language which is compatible with the computer to be used. Simple programmes can be prepared by doctors if they are prepared to spend some time absorbing the principles, but more complicated programmes can often be greatly improved with professional help, for there are many short cuts which enable the programme to be run more quickly. It is the ability to use the computer's characteristics to the full which provides the fascination in programming. However, very few programmes run smoothly the first time and many months are often spent in running and modifying programmes before they are correct in every detail. Even then, mistakes can easily occur during the running of the programme. To minimise these it is necessary to incorporate a series of checks to ensure firstly, that the input data is correct and secondly, that the machine is functioning correctly.

Choice of a computer
The choice of a computer for medical work depends on the type of work to be undertaken. To date, computers have been used for storage and retrieval of patient's records, finance and administration, calculation and presentation of laboratory results and patient monitoring. The type of work will determine the type of input and output units, the size of store and the facilities for tape punching and teletypes which have to be provided either in the central installation or individual departments.

The fascination of using computers in the management of acute illness lies in two possibilities. The first is the computer's ability to perform complex mathematical operations quickly, and then to present the medical personnel with derived data in 'real time'. This is a jargon expression the meaning of which has been stretched to cover the concept that the results are derived fast enough to be acted upon. For example, an intra-arterial needle can provide an accurate trace of pressure, and from it certain factors not immediately obvious, such as the analysis of the upstroke as a measure of cardiac contractility, can be assessed. Unfortunately, the mathematical manipulations on even one heart beat take a considerable time to perform, even with the aid of a desk calculator, certainly too long to influence treatment within the time which may still be available to alter the patient's condition. A computer, however, can be programmed to perform this calculation and present an answer almost on a beat-by-beat basis.

Secondly, the computer can be programmed to store a sequence of such calculations, to make projections concerning a change in state, and to indicate how long will elapse before a certain warning limit will be passed if things continue as they are at present. They are thus able to act as true monitors (*moneo*— I warn) and to alert attendants to the likelihood of some potential emergency in the future.

The use of such on-line facilities throws a heavy load on the installation and requires much more in the way of facilities than off-line usage. It is consequently much more expensive.

REFERENCES

BELLVILLE J.W. & HARA H.H. (1966) Use of analog computers in anesthetic research. *Anesthesiology*, **27**, 70.

CAMPBELL D. & BROWN J. (1963) The electrical analogue of lung. *British Journal of Anaesthesia*, **35**, 684.

COLE J.R., THORNTON J.A., WHELPTON D. & WILSON A.M. (1968) Some applications of analogue computers to teaching. *British Journal of Anaesthesia*, **40**, 373.

MAPLESON W.W. (1964) Mathematical aspects of the uptake, distribution and elimination of inhaled gases and vapours. *British Journal of Anaesthesia*, **36**, 129.

WALD A.A., MURPHY T.W. & MAZZIA V.D.B. (1968) A theoretical study of controlled ventilation. *Biomedical Engineering*, **15**, 237.

FURTHER READING

HOLLINGDALE S.H. & TOOTILL G.C. (1967) *Electronic Computers*. Penguin Books Ltd., Harmondsworth, Middlesex.

6

Spectrophotometry and Other 'Optical' Measurements

Electromagnetic radiations occur in nature at a variety of wavelengths, extending from gamma-rays with a wavelength of less than 0·0001 nanometers (nm), up to radio waves with a wavelength up to thousands of metres. A small part of this spectrum of radiation from about 380 nm to 680 nm can excite the retina and produces a sensation of light. White light consists of a spectrum of colours, extending from the shortest wavelengths, which give the sensation of violet, to the longest visible wavelengths, which excite a sensation of red. Radiations whose wavelengths are just shorter or longer than those of the visible range are designated the ultra-violet and infra-red respectively. Table 6.1 lists the types of radiation and their wavelengths. Wavelengths are measured in a variety of units of length, some of

TABLE 6.1. Spectrum of electromagnetic radiations.

Gamma-rays	<0·01 nm
X-rays	0·01–10 nm
Ultra-violet	10–380 nm
Visible light	380–680 nm
Infra-red	680–6000 nm
Diathermy	Millimetres to metres
Radio waves	Metres upwards

which are hallowed by usage and which may not, therefore, be quickly superseded by the new S.I. units. Of these, the Ångström (Å) is 10^{-10} metres, and therefore 1 nm = 10 Å. Wavelengths used in ultra-violet spectroscopy are frequently expressed in microns (μ) and millimicrons (mμ). Microns are 10^{-6} metres. Millimicrons (10^{-9} m) are therefore the same as nanometres.

The various forms of electromagnetic radiation do not by any means have comparable physical properties. Shorter wavelengths, for example, are not refracted by glass and water, and cannot therefore be focused by these materials. Some wavelengths are considerably absorbed by glass, whereas others may pass freely through optically opaque materials. For the purposes of this chapter, the frequencies of interest lie in the near infra-red (600–6000 nm), within the visible range (380–680 nm) and in the ultra-violet (200–380 nm). From an instrumentation point of view, the behaviour of the whole of this part of the electromagnetic spectrum is broadly similar, and the principles involved in optical instruments are also met with in instruments using solely infra-red or ultra-violet parts of the spectrum. It is often convenient, therefore, to think of them in purely optical terms, although there may be nothing to 'see'.

The basic laws concerning reflection, diffusion, refraction, and absorption of light are fairly complex, but although they are of importance to instrument designers, the successful use of optical instruments does not depend on a knowledge of them, except in the very broadest terms. Thus the absorption of light through a fluid increases exponentially with the distance through the fluid. However, in the completed instrument, the total volume of fluid or the extent of the light path has been fixed by the designer and is usually not under the control of the user. The only physical consideration which should always be borne in mind is that in absorption measurements the degree of absorption is proportional to the quantity of the substance in the light path. In the case of liquids, the quantity is, of course, determined solely by the dimensions of the sample chamber. However, where gases are concerned, changes in pressure will affect the quantity of the substance in the light path, and the amount of absorption will differ from the absorption at atmospheric pressure.

The analysis of mixtures by spectrophotometry can be a very complex process. However, there are instruments of somewhat

3*

simpler construction from which the more complex arrangements are evolved, and which therefore provide a better starting point for discussion.

Simple reflection or transmission instruments
When white light falls on an object which reflects at least some of the radiation in the visible spectrum, we are able to see it. If a surface absorbs all the incident light, it appears black; if it absorbs only certain parts of the spectrum, the reflected light is no longer of a similar composition to the incident light, and the object appears coloured. If the incident light also contains frequencies outside the visible range, but the reflected radiation contains no frequencies within the visible range, the object is, likewise, invisible. For example, many black bodies reflect strongly in the infra-red region, and if a light beam which also contains infra-red radiation falls on a body which reflects nothing in the visible part of the spectrum, it will be invisible to the eye, but will nevertheless be clearly 'seen' by a suitable infra-red detector. Similarly, if a filter between the object and the eye removes all the components to which the retina is sensitive, the object will again be invisible.

Similar considerations apply even when the incident light contains no frequencies in the visible spectrum, since detectors exist which are every bit as specific for particular frequencies as is the human eye. It is thus possible, for example, to detect a change of reflected intensity of one particular wavelength in the presence of others if the conditions can be favourably manipulated. Ideally the substance should only reflect or transmit frequencies for which the detector is specific. However, a similar result could be achieved by inserting a filter which prevented all the light except that of the critical wavelength reaching the detector. Finally, the light source itself could be filtered so that only the desired wavelengths were used.

In a solution which contains semi-absorbent particles, such as red blood corpuscles, the situation is more complex. Some light is reflected back, and some is absorbed in passing through the corpuscles. Both components may then be reflected off other corpuscles and scattered in all directions, including the forward direction. The high degree of transmission through blood is due to the fact that a proportion of the light is subject to multiple reflection and is thus transmitted through the liquid without passing through the solid elements.

A simple instrument which utilises this property is the pulse detector, in which a light source and a photosensitive detector are positioned so that either reflected or transmitted light impinges on the detector. By using a detector which is only sensitive to red light, outside daylight interference is minimised. The rhythmic electrical output can then be used to actuate an intermittent light or sound and can be displayed by a moving pointer, or fed into a ratemeter. Because the fluctuations in electrical signals are proportional to the expansion of the vascular bed by the pulse wave, such instruments are sometimes called, rather erroneously, digital plethysmographs.

Oximeters, which measure the degree of oxygen saturation, are basically constructed in a similar manner, though there are certain complications which make it desirable to defer consideration of them until spectrophotometric measurements have been considered.

SPECTROPHOTOMETERS

Spectrophotometers, oximeters, and some types of gas analysers all contain the same four basic units namely, a light source, filters, a sample chamber and means for detecting the intensity of the radiation. In the case of a spectrophotometer, the first unit contains two sources of electromagnetic radiation, a tungsten lamp for white light and a deuterium source for ultra-violet radiation. The second unit is also more complicated than in some other instruments since it produces radiation with an especially narrow range of wavelengths. Such light, if in the visible spectrum, appears as a pure colour and is therefore termed *monochromatic*. In the spectrophotometer the *monochromator* contains a silica prism, silvered on its back surface. Light is directed into this prism and the emerging light (in the form of a spectrum) is *collimated* by a mirror. By rotating the prism it is possible to

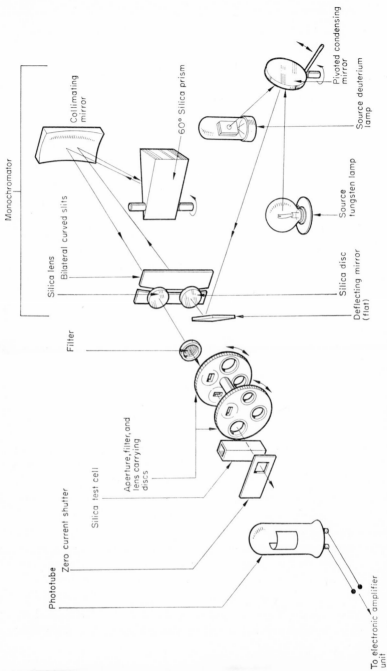

Fig. 6.1. Diagram of a spectrophotometer.

direct a band of the appropriate wavelength through narrow slits. The light can then be further filtered and directed through the sample cell. The optical windows of the sample chamber are usually made of special material, such as quartz, which is translucent to the wavelengths in question. The emergent light which has not been absorbed by the sample is detected quantitatively by the fourth part of the instrument, which is a photoelectric device whose electrical output is proportional to the intensity of light falling upon it. The most common photo-electric devices currently used are semi-conductors (such as cadmium sulphide) which change their resistance when illuminated. They have the great advantage that they only require a low power source and have a high output which is suitable for many recorders without further amplification.

Such a spectrophotometer can be used in two fundamentally different ways. Firstly it can be used to identify an unknown compound. Most substances absorb radiation of different frequencies in a characteristic fashion. Absorption spectra are therefore highly specific. Each absorption band is produced because the energy of certain frequencies of radiation moves orbital electrons from one energy level to another energy level in the same electron shell, or to another shell (see Chapter 7). If the amount of absorption is measured over a whole range of frequencies, the spectrum, which can then be plotted, is characteristic of that substance.

Alternatively, the instrument may be used for quantitative measurements. The absorption spectrum for a compound has one or more frequencies at which absorption is maximal and other frequencies at which it is minimal. Quantitative measurements, at their simplest, involve measuring the amount of absorption at any one frequency, usually the frequency at which absorption is maximal. A linear relationship exists between the quantity of a single substance in a sample and the amount of absorption.

However, the problem is rarely as simple as the assay of the concentration of a pure substance. Frequently, two or more components are present and their absorption spectra overlap, or may interfere with each other so that quite different absorption patterns are formed. Three possible lines of approach are possible. Conceptually, the simplest approach is to perform the measurement at a frequency at which the interfering components have relatively little absorption, compared with the substance of interest. Quite gross variations in the concentration of interfering components will then have little effect on the total absorption, although small changes in concentration of the test substance are easily detected. Unfortunately, in most circumstances, the interference arises from a compound which has considerable absorption at the same wavelength as the substance of interest. In these circumstances, if one knows the absorption of each pure compound at two different wavelengths, and the absorption of the mixture at these wavelengths is measured, the relative concentrations can be derived by solving simultaneous equations. It is necessary to assume that the absorption at the chosen wavelengths is the additive result of the individual absorptions of each component. Accuracy is improved by making the measurements at wavelengths at which one component has a maximal absorption while the other has a minimal absorption, or if these do not coincide, the best compromise between the two. A third approach, which may be appropriate when the components are mixtures of interrelated compounds, is to measure the solution under different sets of conditions which modify the relative proportions of the components, for example, by changing the pH.

Spectrophotometers can also be used to assay enzyme reactions. For example, in the assay of plasma cholinesterase the rate of hydrolysis of the substrate benzoylcholine is measured by the steady increase in transmission of light with time. Rather than measure the actual change in electrical output with a detector, the ubiquitous Wheatstone bridge principle is employed, and a calibrated variable resistor is used to maintain null balance on the bridge.

Oximetry

The same basic principles are employed in oximetry, both absorption and reflection instruments being employed. Here we may

regard the two mutually interfering substances as the reduced
and oxygenated form of haemoglobin. Their relative spectra
are illustrated in Fig. 6.2, and it can be seen that the maximum
difference in the absorption of the two forms of haemoglobin
occurs at a wavelength around 650 nm, while at a frequency
of about 800 nm the *extinction coefficient*, that is to say, the
relative absorption, is the same in both forms. In any mixture
of two components, a point at which the molecular extinction

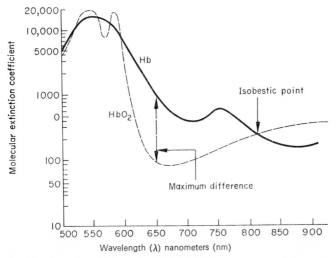

FIG. 6.2. Absorption spectra of reduced (Hb) & oxyhaemoglobin (HbO$_2$).

coefficients are the same is referred to as an *isobestic* point. A
measurement of the light absorbed at the isobestic point is
therefore independent of the degree of oxygenation, and can
be used to standardise the system in terms of the quantity
of haemoglobin, the quantity of plasma proteins, the size of the
sample, and the intensity of the light, etc. If the oximeter is
standardised at this point, and the value is then compared with
a reading taken at 650 nm, the relative difference between the
readings will depend on the degree of oxygen saturation. For
this reason most oximeters have an infra-red source, which
is filtered to provide wavelengths in the appropriate bands.

It is possible to perform oximetry with instruments involving measurement at only one wavelength, but this introduces additional complications. A second cuvette filled with black Indian ink is necessary to provide a zero and compensate for reflection from the glass of the cuvette. The full scale is adjusted by comparing the light from another cuvette filled with a red powder. The conditions must remain stable, since any variation in the wavelength of the light used would destroy the relationship between the relative absorption of the two forms of haemoglobin, and, therefore, more stabilization needs to be built into the lamp heater circuit. A full discussion of the design and operation of various types of oximeters has been given by Reichert (1966).

Additional refinements on this basic pattern have been introduced. For example, non-dispersive gas analysers (Chapter 11) often employ the Luft type of detector in which the radiation emerging from the reference and analysis tubes is absorbed in two gas-filled cells. The difference in temperature between these two cells results in a difference in pressure which is sensed by a diaphragm. By filling the detector chamber with a sample of the gas which is to be measured, its specificity can be increased so that it is only sensitive to the range of frequencies which are of interest. This means that the source and filtering of the infrared light can be less specific. The problem of interference by other compounds with similar absorptions at the relevant frequencies can be similarly overcome by inserting a cell containing the interfering gas in pure form in both the test and reference paths. This ensures that no further absorption can take place if the sample contains the interfering gas.

Cardiac output determination
The use of dye-dilution curves, or time-concentration curves of dye, sensed by an oximeter type of cuvette, is now a common method for measuring cardiac output. The dye which is customarily used now is a form of indocyanine green. This dye has been chosen particularly because its peak absorption occurs at 800 nm, the isobestic point of reduced and oxygenated haemoglobin. Consequently, the sensing device is unaffected by any

changes in the proportion between oxygenated and reduced haemoglobin in the sample during the course of sampling the dye curve. The principle of the determination of cardiac output is discussed in Chapter 9. It is sufficient to notice at this point that any oximeter capable of recording at both 650 and 800 nm is theoretically capable of being used for dye-dilution curves with either Cardiogreen or Coomassie blue (Reichert 1966).

Colorimetry

A large number of biochemical reactions can be performed which lead to the production of a colour the intensity of which is proportional to the biochemical quantity in question. By a suitable selection of filters, it is possible to use a simple light-filter-sample-photoelectric cell system for measuring the intensity of the colour produced.

In all forms of spectrophotometry, oximetry and colorimetry, certain basic problems always arise. There is a need to provide a stable zero, and to have a method of calibrating. It is also usually necessary to provide a reference path in which reagents or blank cells can be inserted, where these influence the total amount of absorption or reflection in the system. Absolute calibration usually depends, in the last analysis, on preparation of accurate standards, or of known dilutions or pure substances. It is the inability to control the physical conditions and the other sources of interference between the light source and the photocell that is responsible for the inadequacy of such devices as ear oximeters.

REFERENCE

REICHERT W.J. (1966) The theory and construction of oximeters. In: *Oxygen Measurements in Blood and Tissues and Their Significance* (eds. Payne J.P. & Hill D.W.). Churchill, London.

FURTHER READING

HILL D.W. (1966) Physics applied to anaesthesia VII. Physical optics, photometry and spectrophotometry. *British Journal of Anaesthesia,* **38**, 964.

7

Measurements Using Radioactive Substances

At the present time, the average anaesthetist has little direct contact with measurements utilising radioisotopes. However, there has recently been a tremendous expansion in the application of radioisotopes to medical problems and an elementary knowledge of the basic principles is now essential.

BASIC CONCEPTS

Atomic structure

All atoms consist of a *nucleus* surrounded by one or more orbital *electrons*. The simplest atom, that of hydrogen, has a nucleus consisting of a single *proton* and one orbiting electron. An electron is negatively charged, whilst the proton is positively charged; to maintain electrical neutrality the number of electrons always equals the number of protons in the pure element. The nucleus of all atoms other than that of hydrogen also contains one or more *neutrons*. These are particles of the same mass as a proton, but which carry no electrical charge. Whilst they add to the weight of a compound, therefore, they have no influence on its chemical behaviour, the latter being determined solely by the number of electrons. Although not strictly accurate, electrons can be thought of as orbiting within well-defined '*shells*'. Each shell is designated by a number, which is called the *principal quantum number*. As one moves from the lightest elements to the heaviest, and the number of orbiting electrons increases, the shells become filled from within outward. A shell is full when it contains $2n^2$ electrons, where n is the principle quantum number. The first shell can therefore, contain two electrons, the second, eight electrons, the third eighteen electrons, and so on. In fact, within each shell, there may be one or more *energy levels* which electrons can take up. If an electron moves from a higher to a lower energy level, either within the shell or by transferring to another shell, then energy is emitted. This is manifested as an emission spectrum. An absorption spectrum is the reverse process. Certain configurations of electrons are relatively unstable, and under appropriate conditions such an atom may gain or lose one or more electrons. As a consequence, it becomes negatively or positively charged, and is then known as an *ion*.

Atoms containing the same number of protons but with different numbers of neutrons are called *isotopes*. Since they have the same number of protons, isotopes also have the same number of electrons, and are, therefore, of course, chemically indistinguishable. Most elements have stable isotopes which do not spontaneously disintegrate. Other isotopes are unstable and their nuclei tend to break down in various ways, and are said to be radioactive. All elements with more than 82 protons seem to be inherently unstable. Some radioactive isotopes exist in nature, but others are only produced artificially in the course of a nuclear reaction or in a cyclotron.

Types of radiation

The disintegration of the nucleus may be accompanied by the emission of particles or energy, or both. *Alpha-radiation* consists of heavy, positively charged particles equivalent to two protons in charge, associated with two further units of mass, making four units of mass in all. They are thus identical with helium nuclei. Emission of an alpha-particle results in the formation of an element with an atomic number two less, and an atomic weight of four less, than the original element.

For example, the initial breakdown of radium leads to the formation of radon

$$^{226}_{88}\text{Ra} \rightarrow {}^{222}_{86}\text{Rn} + \alpha\text{-particle}({}^{4}_{2}\text{He})$$

(The superscripts are the mass number, and the subscripts are the atomic number.)

Although of considerable mass, alpha-particles are not of high velocity and are easily absorbed, even by as little as 0·02 mm of aluminium. However, being doubly charged, they are extremely harmful biologically if once retained in a tissue. They are not used in tracer work. Another type of nuclear disintegration can be thought of as a breakdown of a neutron into a proton and an electron. The electron is ejected as a *beta-particle* and the residual element now has an extra proton, and has become an element with one higher atomic number. For example, lead is converted into bismuth as follows:

$$^{210}_{82}\text{Pb} \rightarrow {}^{210}_{83}\text{Bi} + \beta\text{-particle}({}^{0}_{-1}\beta)$$

Beta-particles emerge with a wide range of energies and are slowed down by collision with electrons of any atoms which are encountered. Beta-radiation is, therefore, also readily absorbed, and the electrons transfer their energy to the local region if administered internally.

In the majority of cases, the emission of the beta-particle is not able to dissipate all the energy that is released during the nuclear rearrangement, and the excess is radiated as *gamma-radiation*, with a characteristic energy quantum. Gamma-radiation is a very shortwave type of electromagnetic radiation, akin to light and radio waves. It is identical with X-radiation (see Table 6.1), and with cosmic radiation, and only the method of production differs. In a nuclear disintegration there is always a characteristic amount of energy released, depending on the original and final configurations, and so the energy levels of gamma-radiation are typical for each type of breakdown. More than one kind of rearrangement may occur, in which case more than one kind of radiation, or more than one level of energy may be characteristic. Highly energetic radiation penetrates more deeply, and is often called 'hard' radiation. Conversely 'soft' radiation has poor penetrating power.

Units of measurement
The fundamental unit is the *curie* (*Ci*) which is defined in terms of the absolute rate of disintegrations. A substance undergoing

3·7 × 10¹⁰ disintegrations per second contains 1 curie of activity. This unit, however, is not of great practical use, because some isotopes emit more than one type of radiation, or more than one particle per disintegration, whilst others emit radiation with only a proportion of the disintegrations. For example, the decay of ^{51}Cr is accompanied by the emission of a gamma-ray in only 8 per cent of the disintegrations. Since it is only the emission either of particles or of gamma-rays which are commonly detected, a measure of emissions is more practical. Such a unit is the *roentgen*, which defines the strength of gamma-rays or X-rays in terms of the amount of ionisation they produce in a cubic centimetre of air. One roentgen can be shown to transfer energy at a rate of about 88 ergs/gramme of air and 97 ergs/gramme of tissue. To incorporate beta-radiation into a measure of radiation potential, the *rad* has been introduced. One rad is the amount of radiation potential from *any* source which transfers 100 ergs/gramme (S.I. units = 0·01 J/kg) to a specified tissue, and is thus approximately equivalent to a roentgen for gamma-radiation.

The energy of any radiation is defined in terms of the electron volt (eV). Most radiations used in medical work have energies between a few keV (thousand electron volts) and 3 MeV (million electron volts).

None of these measurements bear any direct relationship to the number of 'counts' which may be recorded from instruments measuring radioactivity. A radioactive source emits in all directions, and the proportion of its emission which reaches a detecting device depends on the geometric relationship between the two. If the detector is visualised as occupying a finite area on the surface of an imaginary sphere with the source at its centre, the radioactive flux which will impinge on the detector will vary inversely as the square of the radius of that sphere, which is, of course, the distance between the source and the detector. The amount of absorption that takes place between the source and the detector also modifies the amount of the radiation detected, and this depends on the medium through which it is passing. In some cases even a thin perspex window may effectively absorb the radiation. For this reason detectors of quite different designs are needed to match different applications.

Half-life

At any moment the rate of disintegration is dependent on the total number of undisintegrated atoms present. Radioactive decay is therefore exponential, and analogous to such processes as the emptying of the lungs and the metabolism or excretion of many drugs. Any exponential process has a time constant which describes the rate at which the process is proceeding. The time constant (as outlined in Chapter 3) is the time taken to reach 37 per cent of the final value—i.e., 63 per cent of the change is completed in one time constant.

Isotopes differ considerably in the rate at which they disintegrate. The rate varies from hundreds of years in the case of naturally occurring isotopes such as radium, down to only a few seconds for some artificial isotopes, and cannot be altered by any physical or chemical process. It would be quite logical to specify the stability of isotopes by their time constants. In fact, instead of specifying how long it takes for the activity to fall by 63 per cent of its initial value (one time constant), it is customary to specify how long it takes the activity to fall to half its original value. This is actually 0·693 of one time constant. This time is called the *half-life*. It is important to be clear that the half-life is *not* half the time taken for all the activity to disappear. This is an infinite time, since the essence of an exponential decay is that the rate of change is always proportional to the amount of activity present. It will, therefore, take as long for the remaining half of the activity to fall by half again, to one-quarter of the initial value, and as long again to fall to an eighth of the initial value. A knowledge of the half-life therefore enables one to calculate the activity at any future time, once the activity at any time has been determined.

RADIATION DETECTORS

There are many methods of detecting radiation, but for most practical purposes only two types of detectors are commonly used. These are Geiger–Muller and scintillation detectors.

The Geiger counter

This utilises the fact that radiation causes inert gases to ionise. The gas is contained between electrodes, across which a voltage is applied. Ionisation of the gas by radiation produces free electrons and positively charged gas ions, which migrate under the influence of the electric field to produce a current. If the voltage between the electrodes is high and the pressure of gas is low, the electrons, which have negligible mass, are accelerated sufficiently to cause further ionisation when they collide with other gas molecules, and this process is repeated rapidly many times, so that a relatively large electrical signal is produced. A second gas is also included, whose function is to quench any secondary emission caused by the electrons striking the anode.

Geiger counters are very sensitive to beta-radiation (free electrons) but relatively insensitive to gamma-radiation. During the discharge the tube is insensitive until quenching has occurred, and there is, therefore, always a period of lost time, lasting several hundred microseconds, when further ionising radiation will not be detected. For this reason these devices are unsatisfactory for very high counting rates unless corrections for this error are applied.

Scintillation detectors

Radiation will react with certain materials to produce small flashes of light. Such materials are called scintillators or phosphors. For gamma-radiation, the most common detector is a crystal of sodium iodide which produces a tiny flash of light when it interacts with a gamma-ray. Beta-rays can also be detected by scintillation methods, but because they have much less penetrating power the technique is not much employed unless some special indication, such as the need for a fast counting rate, precludes the use of a Geiger counter.

Flashes of light are detected by a semi-transparent photo cathode which emits electrons when exposed to light. A special technique amplifies the feeble current so produced to provide a pulse which is then further amplified before being transmitted along the cable to the rest of the equipment.

Two biologically useful isotopes, ^{14}C and ^{3}H, emit beta-rays of such low energy that most of the emission is absorbed by the sample itself. To overcome this, the sample itself is mixed with a liquid scintillator and the extremely low intensity light flashes are picked up and amplified.

Ancillary equipment

Other equipment is necessary to process the electrical output from either Geiger or scintillation counters. These include a *discriminator*, which rejects signals which are below a critical value, and therefore probably spurious, or a *pulse-height analyser*, which can also reject high-energy cosmic-rays, thus reducing background counting. The pulse-height analyser can also be employed to count a mixture of gamma-ray-emitting isotopes whose emissions occur characteristically at different energy levels; the range of voltages which will be accepted can be adjusted, and this is called the *gate width*.

Pulses which pass the discriminator or pulse height analyser are then fed to the *scaler*, which is a device for counting the pulses. This may be associated with a timer, or more simply, the rate may be measured continuously by a ratemeter.

PROTECTION AGAINST RADIATION HAZARDS

When using radioactive substances, hazards arise in two ways. There may be exposure to radiation during use, or there may be inhalation or ingestion of material which is retained in the body, giving rise to prolonged exposure of some tissues to radiation.

The magnitude of the external hazards depends on the nature of the radiation, the source strength and the duration of exposure. Isotopes emitting only soft beta-radiation constitute less of an external hazard than gamma-emitters. The dose can be controlled by shielding and distance, the dose diminishing inversely as the square of the distance. Ingestion hazards depend on the half-life, on the degree of retention in the body (biological half-life), and whether or not they are concentrated in specific tissues. These factors have been taken into account in a classification of the toxicity of isotopes which is published in the 'Codes of Practice'. Two codes have been formulated which affect medical workers: 'Code of practice for the protection of persons against ionising radiations arising from Medical and Dental Use' (H.M.S.O. 1964) and 'Code of practice for the protection of persons against Ionising Radiations in Research and Teaching' (H.M.S.O. 1964).

In the control of hazards from external radiation, it is of prime importance not to handle isotopes directly. A suitable container or screen should be interposed between the source and any personnel. It is, however, permissible to maintain a sense of proportion. The chief hazard from tracer doses of a few microcuries would be of dropping the lead screening bricks on your foot!

When even 1 μCi amounts of unsealed isotopes are handled, surgical rubber gloves should be worn and washed before being removed. Smoking, eating and drinking, licking labels, etc. should also be avoided.

Isotopes can only be administered to patients by 'Designated Users', and all projects must be approved by an 'Appointed Safety Officer'.

STATISTICS OF COUNTING*

The moment at which any atom of a radioactive source will decay cannot be predicted. It is a random process, and the behaviour of one atom has no influence on the others. There cannot, therefore, be an 'accurate' or 'true' counting rate, but only a mean counting rate. If one were to make many measurements of a radioactive sample and plot the number of times each count was obtained, providing that several hundred counts were recorded on each occasion, the graph would resemble the 'normal' curve, with the peak at the mean counting rate. As such, it is susceptible to statistical inference, as described in Chapter 16. It will be shown that the spread of a normal distribution curve as measured by the standard deviation, is a representation of

* The reading of this section may be delayed until the chapters on statistics have been read.

the variability of the individual results. When variables can take any value (a continuous distribution), the standard deviation is quite independent of the mean. However, when the measurements are counts of events, such as radioactive disintegrations, the two parameters are interrelated. It can be seen intuitively that the more counts are recorded on each occasion, the nearer the result is likely to approach the mean count, and the smaller will be the scatter of results and the smaller the standard deviation. In fact, the variance is equal to the mean count, and the standard deviation is therefore equal to the square root of the mean count. This means that the greater the mean count, the smaller, proportionately, is the standard deviation. For example, a mean count of 100 has a standard deviation of $\sqrt{100}$ or 10, i.e., ± 10 per cent. A mean count of 10,000 has a standard deviation of 100, or ± 1 per cent of the mean.

In practice, one counts a sample once or twice only, and therefore the mean count is not known and so the 'true' standard deviation cannot be calculated. However, if the count is sufficiently large, little error is introduced by using the observed count in place of the mean count. For example, a mean count of 10,000 has a standard deviation of $\sqrt{10,000}$ or 100. We would expect, knowing the properties of the normal curve, that there is a 95 per cent chance that our count is within two standard deviations of the mean count. If our actual count is at the limit, i.e., 10,200, then the standard deviation derived by using this figure would be $\sqrt{10,200}$ or 101 instead of 100. In this number of counts this is a negligible error.

From a knowledge of the normal distribution one can determine the limits within which the 'true' mean count lies at any desired level of probability. A useful approximation is that there is a 95 per cent probability that the answer lies between the limits, counts recorded $\pm 2 \times \sqrt{\text{counts recorded}}$. This is acceptable when the total number of counts exceeds a few hundred.

APPLICATIONS

A wide variety of clinical applications for isotopes have been described. These include measurements of the blood flow in

various organs (Chapter 9), the composition of body compartments (Chapter 10), metabolic turnover studies, and tumour
localization. Radioisotopes are also used therapeutically for
various malignancies. However, such diagnostic and therapeutic
applications are outside the scope of this book.

FURTHER READING

VEALL N. (1969) *Diagnostic Uses of Radioisotopes in Medicine.* Hospital
    Medicine Publications Ltd., London.
HILL D.W. (1968) Physics applied to anaesthesia VIII. Ionising radia-
    tions. *British Journal of Anaesthesia*, **39**, 335.

Part II
Specific Measurements

8

Measurement of Pressure

Pressure is defined as force per unit area. The unit of force in the S.I. system is now the newton (N), this being defined as that force which will accelerate 1 kg at a rate of 1 metre per second per second. It is likely, however, that it will be some time before the unit of pressure 'newtons per square metre' is widely adopted and it is therefore necessary to know the conversion factors for some of the other units. In the older form of the metric system, the unit of force was the dyne (the force which would accelerate 1 gramme at a rate of 1 centimetre per second per second and therefore equal to 10^{-5} N) and pressure was measured in dynes per square centimetre. In the Imperial system pressure was measured in pounds per square inch or pounds per square foot. An alternative method of standardising a pressure measurement is to compare it with the height of a column of liquid, Now,

$$\text{force} = \text{mass} \times g$$

where $g =$ the acceleration due to gravity. But

$$\text{mass} = \text{volume} \times \text{density}$$

Therefore, the force due to a column of liquid

$$= \text{volume} \times \text{density} \times g$$
$$= \text{height} \times \text{cross-sectional area} \times \text{density} \times g$$

But

$$\text{pressure} = \text{force per unit area}$$

Therefore, the pressure exerted by a column of liquid is given by

$$\frac{\text{height} \times \text{cross-sectional area} \times \text{density} \times g}{\text{cross sectional area}} = \text{height} \times \text{density} \times g$$

g is, for all practical purposes, a constant (980 cm or 32 feet per second per second) so that the pressure exerted by a column of fluid is linearly related to its height and density. For this reason it is essential to specify the liquid used in the manometer. Conversion factors for pressures are shown in Table 8.1.

TABLE 8.1. Conversion factors for units of pressure.

S.I. unit	Old metric	Imperial	Water column	Mercury column	mbar	bar
Newton/ m^2	Dynes/ cm^2	Pounds force/ in^2	mmH_2O	mmHg		
1	10	0·000145	0·1020	0·0075	10^{-2}	10^{-5}
9·8064	98·0638	0·00143	1	0·0735	0·0980	0·000098
133·3224	1333·2240	0·0194	13·5955	1	1·3332	0·0013

1 atmosphere = 101,325 N/m² = 1013250 dynes/cm² = 760 torr.

The torr is now tending to replace the mmHg in very accurate work, since it is independent of such variables as the density of mercury at different temperatures and pressures.

Liquid manometers

Two basic types of liquid manometer are used, the first yielding absolute values of pressure (Fig. 8.1) and the second, pressure relative to atmospheric pressure (Fig. 8.2). The first type of manometer is usually used for the measurement of atmospheric pressure (barometer) and pressures below atmospheric. Atmospheric pressure will support a column of mercury 76 cm high, hence the pressure is about 10^6 dynes per cm^2 or just over one bar. Since the density of mercury is 13·6 × the density of water, 1 atmosphere is equivalent to a column of water 1033 cm (33·9 feet) high.

When using U-tube manometers it is important to remember that the pressure is given by the difference in height between the two menisci, and not the distance of each meniscus from the zero point. In single-tube manometers the height of the column is measured from the meniscus in the reservoir. If the surface area of the reservoir is large in comparison with the cross-sectional area of the tube, the level of the meniscus in the reservoir will vary little in relation to the movement of the meniscus in the tube. It is therefore possible to fix a permanent scale on the tube without introducing too much error. This is

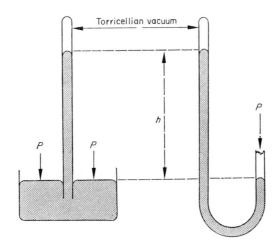

FIG. 8.1. Liquid manometer yielding absolute pressure (e.g. barometer).

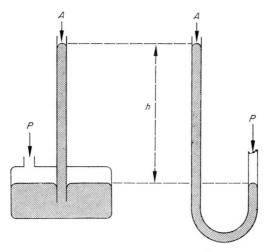

FIG. 8.2. Liquid manometer giving pressures above atmospheric.

4

a great convenience in certain situations, for example when measuring blood pressure with the sphygmomanometer.

The sensitivity of liquid manometers can be increased in a number of ways. The most obvious method is to use a liquid of low density, such as alcohol or liquid paraffin. Another method is to incline the tube so that the vertical movement of the meniscus is amplified (Fig. 8.3). In such an *inclined plane* manometer great care must be taken to level the baseplate accurately before taking a reading. Yet another way of increasing sensitivity is

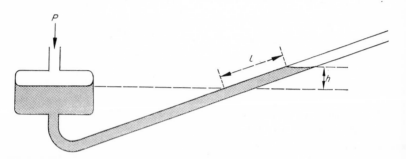

FIG. 8.3. Inclined plane manometer.

to use a differential liquid manometer (Fig. 8.4). Two non-miscible liquids of slightly different density are placed in opposing limbs of a U-tube, the quantities of each liquid being adjusted so that a meniscus is formed close to the top of one limb of the U. If the pressure to be measured is now applied to this limb the meniscus will be displaced downwards. If the two reservoirs at the top have a large cross-sectional area compared with the U-tube a large movement of the meniscus can occur without there being much difference in height between the fluid levels in the two reservoirs. If this slight difference in height is ignored it can be seen that the movement of the meniscus will be inversely related to the difference in density between the two liquids:

$$\Delta P = h(d_1 - d_2)g$$

where ΔP = the pressure difference to be measured

h = the movement of the meniscus

d_1 and d_2 are the densities of the two liquids

Therefore,

$$h = \frac{\Delta P}{(d_1 - d_2)g}$$

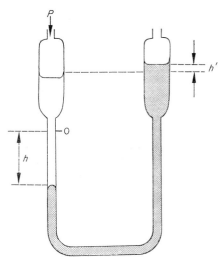

FIG. 8.4. Differential liquid manometer. h' is small in relation to h because of the difference in diameter between the manometer tube and reservoirs.

Hence, sensitivity can be increased by using two liquids of very similar density.

The sensitivity of a manometer can be decreased by filling the closed end of the U-tube with a gas (Fig. 8.5). The movement of the meniscus is then governed by the height and density of the liquid column and the balancing pressure exerted by the compressed gas. The latter can be calculated by the application of Boyle's Law. This type of manometer is used for measuring such high pressures that the length of the mercury column would become unmanageable (see page 96 and Fig. 8.14).

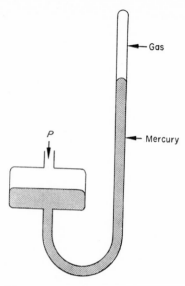

FIG. 8.5. Liquid manometer for measurement of high pressures.

Bourdon gauge

This type of manometer is usually used for measuring high pressures but can also be adapted for the measurement of temperature (Chapter 13) and flow (page 125).

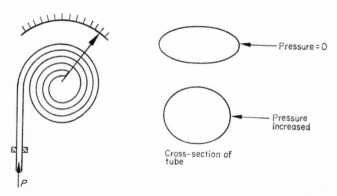

FIG. 8.6. Bourdon gauge.

The gauge consists of a coiled tube which is flattened in cross-section (Fig. 8.6). One end of the coil is anchored to the case and connected to the source of pressure, whilst the other end is closed and attached to a mechanism which drives the pointer on the dial. The application of pressure to the inside of the tube causes the cross-section to become more circular. This causes the coiled tube to straighten. Since one end is fixed, the other unwinds, and so moves the pointer across the dial.

Aneroid gauge

For more moderate pressures a metal bellows is often used to sense the pressure. Expansion of this bellows is detected by a

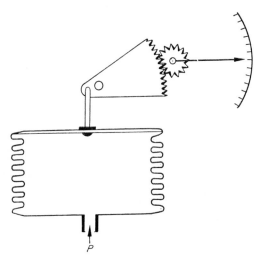

FIG. 8.7. Aneroid gauge.

lever mechanism which amplifies the movement and drives the pointer across the scale (Fig. 8.7). An aneroid bellows can be seen working in the 'Bosun' warning device. When a failure of oxygen line pressure allows the bellows to collapse, an electrical contact and a gas valve on a shaft attached to the bellows are both actuated.

Diaphragm gauge

Most physiological pressure measurements are now made by sensing the movement of an elastic diaphragm. This movement can be sensed directly or converted into electrical energy for subsequent processing and display.

Direct sensing can be carried out by attaching a thread to the centre of the diaphragm, the other end being connected to a writing arm. This arrangement is not very accurate and possesses

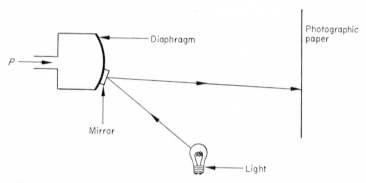

FIG. 8.8. Use of a mirror to sense the movement of a transducer diaphragm.

marked inertia. An improved method of sensing the movement of the diaphragm (used by many of the early physiological workers) is shown in Fig. 8.8. A small mirror is attached to one side of the diaphragm. When the diaphragm is stretched by the application of pressure it becomes curved and the mirror is rotated. The displacement of the mirror is recorded by reflecting a beam of light onto photographic paper. Great sensitivity is possible since the light path can be lengthened by reflecting it back and forth between fixed mirrors.

The *indirect methods* of sensing the movement of a diaphragm involve the conversion of the mechanical energy imparted to the diaphragm into electrical energy. This is then processed and fed to a display unit or recorder. The mechanical energy is said to be *transduced* into electrical energy and the instrument which carries out this process is termed a *transducer*.

Physical principles of transducers

Many methods of sensing the movement of the diaphragm have been suggested in the past but the following are those most commonly used in apparatus available today.

Optical. The back of the diaphragm is silvered and a beam of light is reflected on to a photo-electric cell. As the diaphragm

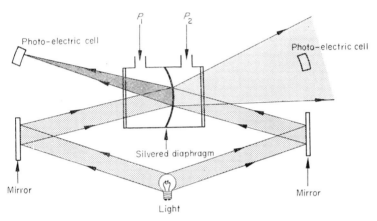

Fig. 8.9. Optical defocusing manometer.

is pressurised the silvered surface becomes convex. The intensity of light sensed by the photo-electric cell is reduced and its electrical output falls. If both sides of the diaphragm are silvered and two photo-electric cells are used the instrument becomes even more sensitive (Fig. 8.9).

Strain gauge. This depends on the fact that when a wire is stretched or compressed it undergoes a change in resistance (Fig. 8.10). To improve the sensitivity the wires are arranged so that one pair of wires is stretched while another pair is compressed. The change in resistance is measured by incorporating the wires in a Wheatstone bridge system (see Chapter 3). The voltage change which appears across the bridge is proportional to the change in resistance. Signals are of the order of 20–50 μV/mmHg pressure change. Much greater sensitivity can be achieved by the use of silicon strain gauge elements. Indeed, in some transducers the output is sufficient to drive a recorder directly.

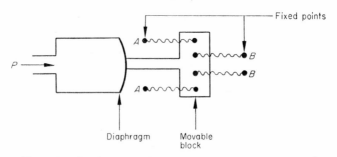

Fig. 8.10. Strain gauge. Points A, A and B, B are fixed.

Capacitance. The diaphragm of the pressure transducer is used as one plate of a capacitor, the second plate being fixed. Movement of the diaphragm varies the distance between the plates, and this varies the charge which can be carried by the capacitor. This is sensed by an appropriate electronic circuit. This type of transducer can be made very sensitive but it is also much affected by ambient temperature variation. This renders it relatively unstable.

Inductance. The inductance of a coil can be varied by changing the position of a core of magnetic material lying within the magnetic field of the coil (Fig. 8.11). The magnetic core is attached to the diaphragm and the inductance of the coil is

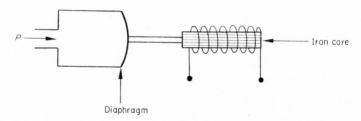

Fig. 8.11. Variable inductance transducer.

measured by making it part of a Wheatstone bridge circuit which is energised by an alternating current.

A more common form of inductance transducer is that employing a differential transformer (Fig. 8.12). The core is placed between the two secondary windings of a transformer. When it is situated symmetrically between them the a.c. voltage induced in the secondary coils is equal in magnitude but opposite in phase. There is therefore zero output. If the core is now displaced by

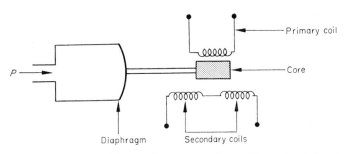

Fig. 8.12. Differential transformer transducer. The output signal appears across the secondary coils.

movement of the diaphragm the voltage in one coil will exceed that in the other and an output voltage will appear at the terminals. If the core is moved in the opposite direction the output will be equal in voltage but opposite in phase. By using a phase-sensitive rectifier (which changes the a.c. signals to d.c.) an appropriate d.c. voltage will be produced.

MEASUREMENT OF INTRAVASCULAR PRESSURES

The ventricular rate and the arterial and venous pressure are the aspects of cardiovascular function that are most frequently monitored in anaesthesia. The relative ease with which these measurements are made should not obscure the fact that they are the resultant of several variables and only indirectly related to cardiac output and tissue perfusion. Instruments are available for measuring arterial blood pressure indirectly, but if an accurate measurement, a tracing of the waveform or a continuous

4*

recording is required, then it is generally necessary to measure the pressure within the lumen of an artery directly.

A rough measurement of venous pressure can be made by examination of the neck veins or by elevating the arm and observing the height at which the veins collapse. An accurate measurement of central venous pressure requires cannulation of the superior vena cava or right atrium.

DIRECT METHODS

Liquid manometers

Water or mercury manometers can only be used to measure mean pressures in the circulatory system, since their inertia is high. Despite this limitation their simplicity is a great attraction. Mercury manometers must be connected to the blood vessel with a catheter containing saline, they are difficult to sterilise and there is always the risk of mercury emboli. Although widely used in laboratories, they are, therefore, rarely used clinically. Saline manometers are much easier to use and are ideal for venous pressure monitoring.

Arterial pressure. This can be recorded on a U-tube mercury manometer with limbs about 35 cm in length. The arrangement shown in Fig. 8.13 is often used. If an open-ended saline manometer is used the length of the vertical limb required becomes unmanageable. An alternative plan is to use a saline manometer with a closed tube and a compressed gas bubble (Fig. 8.14). This needs to be calibrated initially but remains accurate thereafter, provided that ambient temperature does not change too much (Fink 1963). An aneroid blood-pressure manometer gauge may also be used for arterial pressure recording, providing the bellows is sterilised and no liquid is allowed to enter the gauge (Fig. 8.15) (Zorab 1969).

Venous pressure. Saline manometers are ideal for measuring venous pressure (Sykes 1963). A simple T-piece system is all that is required (Fig. 8.16). The catheter must be inserted into a central vein (via median cubital, subclavian, femoral, external or internal jugular venepuncture or cut-down) and there should

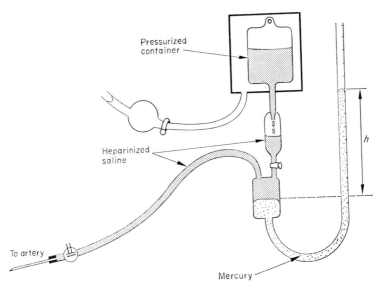

FIG. 8.13. Mercury manometer arranged for blood-pressure measurement.

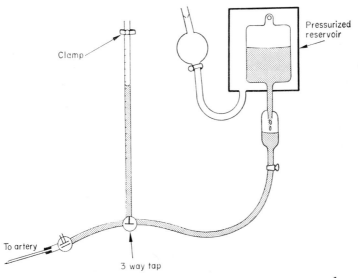

FIG. 8.14. Saline manometer adapted for arterial-pressure recording (Fink 1963).

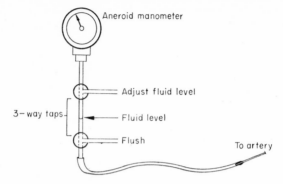

FIG. 8.15. Aneroid gauge used for arterial-pressure recording (Zorab 1969).

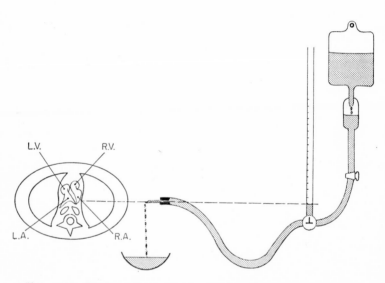

FIG. 8.16. Hydrostatic method of adjusting venous pressure manometer zero. The manometer tube is lowered and this, and the patient limb, are filled with saline whilst the end of the patient limb is held opposite the mid-axillary line. The manometer limb is then raised slowly whilst the saline is allowed to run out of the patient limb. The level of saline in the manometer limb remains at the level of the outlet from the patient limb; the manometer tube is raised until the saline meniscus is at zero and is then clamped to the dripstand.

be a dependent loop of tubing between the manometer and venous catheter to minimise the risk of air embolus. The zero reference point should be the right atrium, the surface markings being the junction of a line running in the coronal plane half-way between the xiphoid and the dorsum of the body and a line drawn at right-angles to the fourth interspace where it meets the sternum (Winsor & Burch 1945) (Fig. 8.17). The zero point on the manometer scale can be adjusted to be in the same horizontal plane by the use of a stick with attached spirit level or

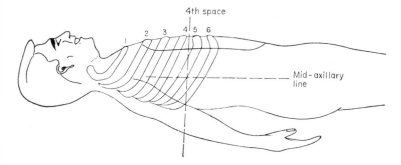

FIG. 8.17. Zero reference point for venous pressure measurement.

by an optical sight. Alternatively a hydrostatic method may be used (Fig. 8.16). An arm which drops down at right-angles to the drip stand provides another simple method of setting the zero (Fig. 8.18).

In clinical practice it is often convenient to use the junction of manubrium and sternum as the anatomical reference point. It must, however, be remembered that venous pressure measured from this reference point will be 5–10 cm lower than that recorded using the true reference point at the atrial level (Debrunner & Bühler 1969). Since the normal venous pressure is 0–10 cm H_2O when referred to the atrium, negative values will often be obtained when the manubriosternal junction is used as the zero level.

It must be emphasised that errors may arise in venous pressure measurement if the catheter is not in a central vein or if the catheter becomes blocked by clot or by impaction against the vein wall. A reading should only be accepted when respiratory swings are clearly visible. Falsely high readings are also obtained

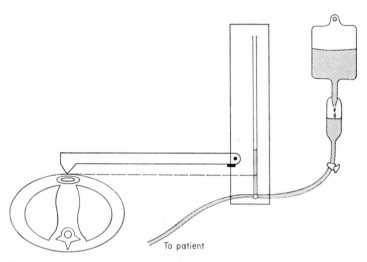

FIG. 8.18. Use of a hinged arm to set the manometer zero. The arm folds back into the stand when not in use. The manubriosternal junction is being used as a reference point.

when the tip of the catheter slips into the right ventricle or the end of the manometer tube becomes blocked (e.g. by a wet cotton wool filter).

Pressure transducers

Although it is possible to construct a pressure transducer which is small enough to be placed within the lumen of the vessel, the routine technique is to connect the lumen of the vessel to the pressure transducer by a fluid-filled catheter. The fluid and the diaphragm of the transducer then constitute a system which will undergo Simple Harmonic Motion (S.H.M.). The fluid and the mass of the diaphragm constitute the oscillating mass, and the diaphragm is the spring. Such a system can only record the pressure and waveform accurately if certain physical conditions are satisfied.

Physical principles governing the use of pressure transducers

Resonant frequency. The first condition governing successful reproduction of a pressure waveform is that the natural or resonant frequency of the system must be higher than the oscillation it is trying to follow.

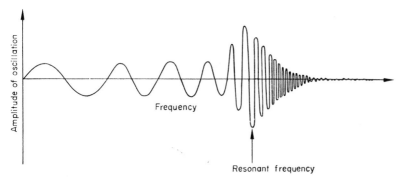

FIG. 8.19. Amplitude of oscillation of a diaphragm in a pressure transducer as the applied frequency is increased. At the undamped natural frequency (resonant frequency) the amplitude is maximal but at higher frequencies the diaphragm fails to follow the applied force.

Any system capable of oscillating in S.H.M. has a natural frequency of oscillation if it is set in motion and there are no forces opposing the motion (Fig. 8.19). Its value is determined by the general formula

$$\text{undamped frequency} \propto \frac{1}{2\pi}\sqrt{\frac{S}{M}}$$

where S is the stiffness of the spring and M is the oscillating mass. In the present discussion these factors refer to the stiffness of the diaphragm and the mass of fluid in the catheter and transducer.

From this equation it would appear that the natural frequency would be highest when the diaphragm was as stiff as possible, and the oscillating mass was as small as possible. Furthermore, since the fluid in both the catheter and the transducer is part of the mass, it would seem that a small volume should be contained in both. Unfortunately, the mass term cannot be viewed as merely the sum of the various oscillating masses. The essence of an oscillating system is the continual interchange between energy in two forms; in this case it is between the kinetic energy of the mass in motion, and the potential energy of the deformed spring. Now, the kinetic energy of the mass in motion is mass times the *square* of the velocity, so that it takes more energy to make any given mass of fluid oscillate in a narrow tube than in a wider tube, because it has to reach a higher velocity in the narrow tube. (This ignores the effect of friction, which will be discussed later.) Since the velocity is inversely proportional to the cross-sectional area of the catheter, the mass term in the equation must be adjusted by dividing the mass of each part of the system by the square of the cross-sectional area of that part. When this is done it is found that the mass in the catheter is the only significant mass in the system. (See the appendix at the end of the chapter for a worked example.)

The stiffness of the diaphragm of a transducer is usually expressed as its volume displacement, in $mm^3/100$ mmHg. This is, in fact, the reciprocal of stiffness. The formula for the natural frequency of the catheter–transducer system is therefore

$$\text{natural frequency} \propto \frac{1}{2\pi}\sqrt{\frac{\pi r^2}{l \times E}}$$

where E is the volume displacement of the transducer and l and r are the length and radius of the catheter.

To obtain an accurate tracing of a complex waveform, one should ideally be able to reproduce every frequency contained in it. In practice, as long as the system can follow ten times the fundamental frequency, no noticeable distortion results. For a pulse rate of 180/min this means a system able to respond to frequencies up to 30 Hz.

Damping. There is, however, a second factor which must be considered. Although we have considered the natural frequency, in practice the system always contains a fluid which is subject to frictional resistance when it moves and this damps the system, i.e. prevents it reaching its final position immediately.

An oscillating system which, when displaced, returns exactly to its former position without overshoot or oscillation, is said to be critically damped (Fig. 8.20b). Such a system is too damped

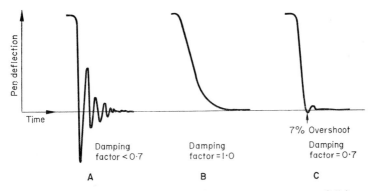

FIG. 8.20. The response of a transducer to a square-wave fall in pressure produced by bursting a rubber balloon pressurised with air. (a) undamped, (b) critically damped, (c) damping 70 per cent of critical. Damping factor is the degree of damping expressed as a fraction of critical damping.

to record rapid oscillations. Underdamping also seriously distorts the waveform. In an underdamped system applied oscillations which are near the natural frequency of the recording system become grossly amplified (Fig. 8.20A). As damping is increased this over-reaction becomes less marked, and when it becomes about 70 per cent of critical the amplitude of the response is close to that of the applied force at frequencies up to two-thirds of the natural frequency of the system (Fig. 8.20C).

Phase shift. Damping also causes a time delay or phase shift between the applied force and the response. For a complex wave it is essential that all the components should be delayed by the same amount of time and this means that the delay must be proportionately increased as frequency increases. This only applies when damping is about 70 per cent of critical (Fig. 8.21).

When faithful reproduction of frequencies up to 30 Hz is necessary the system should have a natural frequency of at least
45 Hz. If the natural frequency is below this the waveform will
be distorted, and the values of systolic and diastolic pressure
may not be accurate. The mean blood pressure will still be
reasonably correct, since this is usually obtained by deliberately
applying overdamping.

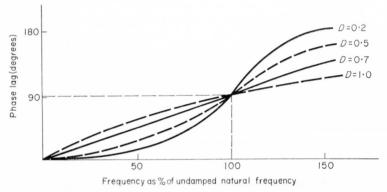

FIG. 8.21. Relation of phase shift to damping.

Although it is possible to calculate the theoretical specification
of the system from the foregoing considerations, such values are
usually not obtained in practice because of the presence of air
bubbles. As the pressure changes from systolic to diastolic the
bubbles change in volume, and with even quite a small bubble
the volume of saline that flows in and out of the catheter in
response to this volume change may be greater than the volume
change due to the displacement of the transducer diaphragm.
Since this extra flow has to take place during the same time
interval, the velocity of the flow is increased, and this increases
the effective mass of the system. This has two effects. It lowers
the natural frequency of the system, and may bring it below the
frequencies which are being applied; and it increases the damping. These effects do not depend on the bubble being in the
catheter, and are just the same if it is on the side wall of the

transducer. It is of the greatest practical importance, therefore, to avoid bubbles anywhere in the system. In the most stringent applications boiled saline is used to flush the catheter and transducer system.

It may be mentioned here that recent developments in transducer design have eliminated many of the problems associated with the mass of fluid and the diameter of the catheter. High-sensitivity transducers can now be made with such a low volume displacement that it is possible to have a natural frequency in the region of 200 Hz. With such a transducer the significant frequencies at ordinary pulse rates are less than 10 per cent of the natural frequency. Under these conditions, amplitude and phase distortions are negligible, provided that bubbles do not significantly lower the natural frequency.

Adjustment of damping
Damping of the system can be increased both hydrostatically and electrically. It can be increased hydrostatically by inserting an additional constriction in the system, or by allowing the velocity of flow in the catheter to rise by inserting a compliant tube into the system. Electrical damping can be accomplished by passing the electrical signal arising from the moving diaphragm through frequency selective circuits. It must be emphasised, however, that manipulation of electronic controls cannot put back frequencies that were lost on their way to the transducer. Regular flushing to prevent clotting and to remove air bubbles is essential.

It has already been explained that problems of damping can be minimised by the use of a correctly balanced catheter–transducer system or by the use of a transducer with a very low volume displacement. If the natural frequency of the transducer is high in relation to the frequencies being recorded, the amount of damping makes little difference and there are only small errors. Such conditions are not often achieved in practice. When the natural frequency is closer to the frequencies applied, only a critically damped system will be accurate. When the natural frequency is so low that important harmonics of the pressure wave correspond with it, overdamped systems produce a smaller error than underdamped ones. Since it is difficult to measure, still less control, the damping, it is common practice to increase the damping if the record looks 'spiky', the assumption being that this is due to the higher frequencies being near the resonant frequency.

This approach, while pragmatic, is making the best of what may be a very bad job. If accuracy is important one must make some evaluation of the frequency response in the prevailing conditions. This can be done by observing the response to a sudden step-wise change. If a trace is made by recording the static pressure in a balloon which is then burst with a hot wire, there will be an immediate (square wave) drop in pressure. When the system is very underdamped there is a large overshoot. When it is overdamped the response is sluggish and the new value of the pressure is reached only gradually, and when damping is ideal the first overshoot is about 6–7 per cent of the initial step change (Fig. 8.20c). It is desirable to aim to exceed this figure and then apply further damping electrically.

CHOICE OF APPARATUS FOR INTRAVASCULAR PRESSURE MEASUREMENT

In order to obtain a high natural frequency, designers of transducers for arterial pressure recording have been developing stiffer and stiffer diaphragms, with smaller volume displacements.

Transducers with a volume displacement of $0 \cdot 01$ mm^3/100 mmHg seem to have reached practicable limits. The compressibility of saline is such that for a pressure change of 100 mmHg a 1 ml chamber would take up nearly $0 \cdot 006$ mm^3, just over half the volume displacement. Unless the volume of the chamber can be considerably reduced, any further increase in stiffness can yield little dividend in terms of natural frequency. This is because the major factors determining the characteristics of the system will now be those produced by the saline moving down the catheter to supply the volume changes of the saline in the transducer chamber. For this reason when the highest frequency response is required transducers are now placed at the distal end of the catheter, within the lumen of the blood vessel itself.

Whatever the system, a stiffer diaphragm has to be paid for by a reduced sensitivity of the system. A stiff diaphragm must result in smaller movement for a given pressure change, and no matter what method is used to sense that movement, a smaller change of that quantity will result. A high frequency response, and a sensitive system, are therefore mutually incompatible characteristics.

Venous pressure measurements require high sensitivity, but very little high-frequency capability, and transducers with a high volume displacement should be used. If the shape of the wave-form is of importance, arterial tracings need a high frequency response, and a really low volume displacement is essential. If the shape of the waveform is not of crucial importance, and it is only desired to record the systolic and diastolic pressures, a flat response up to 10 Hz will give figures within 5 per cent of the correct figure, despite amplitude and phase distortion.

INDIRECT METHODS FOR ARTERIAL PRESSURE

The simplest method of taking blood pressures is with the Riva-Rocci cuff and auscultation of the Korotkov sounds (Fig. 8.22). Although this method is in everyday use, the accuracy

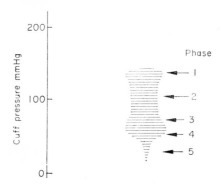

FIG. 8.22. Korotkov sounds.

obtained is very variable and depends on several factors: the interpretation of the sounds themselves, the width of the cuff, and the size and composition of the arm.

The Korotkov sounds

The mechanism of production of the Korotkov sounds is not fully agreed, but a reasonable conceptual model is that turbulent flow makes the artery wall vibrate excessively and this is more or less amplified by a resonance 'ringing' of tissues of the arm. The artery wall vibrates excessively between systolic and diastolic pressures because the vessel under the cuff has no transmural pressure at some stage during the beat. The sound contains an initial high-frequency component due to the turbulence, and this is lost during Phase IV. The low-frequency component is about 50–60 Hz and can be reproduced by tapping any part of the arm. Systolic pressure is taken to be the cuff pressure when the sound is first heard. Some flow actually occurs before this but has insufficient energy to create a sound. Indirect measurements of systolic pressure, therefore, always give a lower figure than simultaneous intra-arterial manometric measurements, and this discrepancy is increased by using too large a cuff. This is presumably because, when an artery is compressed, the pulse wave is retarded, and it needs a bigger flow before the wave traverses the compressed segment with sufficient turbulence to produce a sound. The Korotkov sounds are first heard, therefore, well below the onset of first flow. Narrow cuffs, on the other hand, give a reading which is too high. Tissue pressure is less than cuff pressure under the outermost 5 cm of the cuff in adults, and cuffs must be wider than 10 cm before the cuff pressure is applied to the artery. A more useful relationship exists between required cuff width and arm size. The American Heart Association (1967) recommends a cuff width of 13 cm or 20 per cent greater than the diameter of the arm. Irvine (1968) recommends that a 12 cm cuff should be used for arms of less than 28 cm girth, and a 14 cm cuff for arms bigger than this. A range of smaller sizes should be used in infants and children. A satisfactory rough guide for arms of normal girth is that the cuff should equal one-third to one-half the distance between elbow and shoulder. Errors produced by inappropriate cuff sizes are greater in hypertensive subjects.

As the cuff pressure is reduced, the Korotkov sounds become muffled (Phase IV) and eventually disappear (Phase V). The onset of Phase IV is associated with the loss of the high-frequency component and is believed to indicate the onset of continuous flow. However, its recognition depends a good deal on subjective interpretation.

The American Heart Association (1967) has recommended that Phase IV should be taken as the diastolic end-point. This is defined as a sudden muffling of the Korotkov sounds, or a sudden drop in frequency below 60 Hz. They found that the Phase IV end-point overestimated the intra-arterial diastolic pressure by 5–10 mm Hg but that this was a systematic error. Although Phase V has a better mean correlation with the true diastolic pressure it is subject to larger random errors. Both auscultation points give, on average, an over-estimate of the diastolic pressure.

Instrumental methods for taking both pressures by using the Korotkov sounds have been fraught with difficulties, and have been largely abandoned. The systolic signal (Phase I) is suitable in itself, being an abrupt change, but both Phase IV and V are associated with gradually changing signals. Both are extremely sensitive to interference by noise; any bang on the patient or the microphone will be interpreted as a signal, as will movement of the microphone on the arm.

Other cuff methods
Systolic pressure is most amenable to instrumentation, since the onset of flow can be detected in a variety of ways (Crul 1962). There is the further advantage that the cuff can be placed round the finger instead of the arm. This can allow continuous inflation of the cuff, since there is no muscle to become ischaemic. The cuff and detector should be separated by at least one joint. It becomes particularly important to consider the position of the cuff in relation to the heart when using finger cuffs for the hydrostatic pressure between the cuff and the heart contributes to the

pressure in the vessels in the finger. When the arm is hanging and the subject is erect, the blood pressure in the finger will be 30–40 mm Hg higher than when the finger is at heart height. The commonest pulse detector is a photo-electric cell, sensitive to a change in either transmission or reflection of red light. The reflection type can be made very small, attached almost anywhere, and is less prone to interference from incident light. Another common detector system is a partially inflated second cuff; expansion of the part under the second cuff is detected by the movement of air in and out of the cuff which cools a thermistor. Piezo-electric crystals are also suitable for detecting finger expansion. Unfortunately, most of these methods become inaccurate or cease to function when the blood pressure is low or the periphery is vasoconstricted.

A version of a second cuff detector is used in the von Recklinghausen oscillotonometer (Fig. 8.23). There are two different models of oscillotonometer in clinical use today, namely the

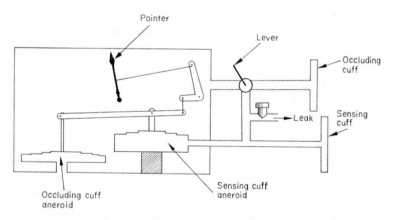

FIG. 8.23. Diagram of oscillotonometer.

Scala Alternans and the Scala Alternans Altera, although a number of other instruments have been used in the past (Barry 1950). The two models are of slightly different design, but work on similar principles. The 'Altera' is the only model in current production. Two partially overlapping cuffs are placed around the upper arm, care being taken that the occluding cuff is placed uppermost. The occluding cuff is connected to the interior of the instrument through a spring-loaded tap, whilst the sensing cuff is connected directly to an aneroid chamber. One side of this chamber is fixed to the casing of the instrument, whilst the other is attached to a short arm which acts as the fulcrum for a longer arm. One end of the long arm is attached to a second aneroid chamber (which is connected to atmosphere), whilst the other is attached to a lever movement which causes the needle on the dial to rotate.

When the hand bulb is squeezed air is pumped into both cuffs and into the main chamber of the oscillotonometer. This is continued until the pressure exceeds the systolic pressure. The valve situated on the casing is then slightly opened and the spring-loaded lever is pulled towards the operator. The movement of the lever connects the occluding cuff and main chamber to the valve and so allows the pressure in the occluding cuff to fall in a controlled fashion. The movement of the lever also isolates the sensing cuff and its aneroid, although there is still a connection between the inside of the aneroid and the main chamber through a small pinhole in the diaphragm. This hole maintains approximate equilibrium between the pressure in the two chambers but is not large enough to affect the pressure changes in the sensing chamber resulting from the pulsatile changes in pressure in the sensing cuff.

As the pressure in the occluding cuff and main chamber falls, a point is reached at which blood starts to flow into the segment of artery under the sensing cuff. The pulsations of the artery under the sensing cuff are transmitted to the aneroid chamber and so move the fulcrum of the long arm. This movement is transmitted to the needle, so that large oscillations suddenly appear on the dial as the upper cuff pressure falls below systolic. When these pulsations become apparent the spring-loaded lever is released. This action once again connects the sensing cuff aneroid to the main chamber, thus equalising the pressure on both sides of the sensing aneroid diaphragm and allowing it to return to its normal resting position. When this position has been reached the reading on the dial will be related solely to the position of the occluding cuff aneroid diaphragm, and the systolic pressure can therefore be accurately read off the scale. The lever is then depressed once more and the leak is allowed to continue until the pulsations recorded on the dial diminish. The lever is released and the diastolic pressure is read. The cuffs and chamber are then returned to atmospheric pressure by opening the quick-release valve close to the bulb.

It can be seen that the instrument utilises the same underlying mechanisms as other indirect methods of blood-pressure measurement. It is therefore prone to the same errors, namely recording the systolic pressure below its true value and the diastolic above. It tends to be least accurate at high pressures, and low pulse pressures. It performs at its best in the presence of moderate hypotension associated with peripheral vasodilation. Fortunately, these are the conditions in which it is most often used.

The triple cuff method
This method, originated by de Dobbeleer (1963) and often called the phase shift method, relies on the fact that the pulse wave travels more slowly through a partially compressed artery. The method has proved to be reliable enough for automation and the commercially available instrument (Godart haemotonograph) which employs this principle has proved to be the only indirect instrument which works at all satisfactorily in all situations. Three cuffs are used in one harness. The first two overlap, and extend for 14 cm; the third is separate and measures only 1 cm. The complete cuff assembly is blown up above systolic pressure and deflated automatically at about 3 mm/sec. The first pulsation which traverses the upper cuff system expands the third cuff, and expels a small quantity of air. This is sensed by a thermistor, and this signal is used to lock a gauge at systolic pressure and to actuate the upper cuff sensing system. The latter consists of another sensing thermistor which is in direct line with an outlet from the upper cuff (Fig. 8.24). An outlet from the

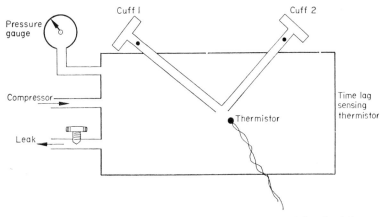

Fig. 8.24. Diastolic pressure sensing system: principle of triple cuff method of indirect measurement of blood pressure.

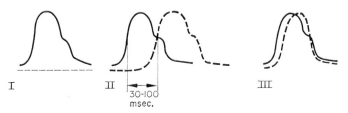

Fig. 8.25. Tracings of signals from thermistors inserted in leads to cuff 1 (solid line) and cuff 2 (broken line). I. Above systolic pressure no pressure wave reaches cuff 2. II. Between systolic and diastolic pressure, there is a delay of 30–100 milliseconds between the pressure wave at cuff 1 and its arrival at cuff 2. III. At diastolic pressure, there is virtually no delay, and both signals occur together. Above systolic pressure, the thermistor is rhythmically cooled by puffs of air from cuff 1. There is no pulsation from cuff 2. Between systolic and diastolic pressure, the thermistor is rhythmically cooled by puffs of air from cuff 1; the puff of air from cuff 2 comes 30–100 milliseconds later, when air flow from cuff 1 is minimal. At diastolic pressure and below, both puffs of air arrive simultaneously, and the air-stream from cuff 1 is diverted by the air-stream from cuff 2. The thermistor is not cooled, and no rhythmic signal is generated.

second cuff faces across the line of exit from cuff 1. During the passage of the pulse wave a puff of air from the upper cuff cools the thermistor, which generates an alternating signal. Owing to the delay caused by the arterial compression, the puff from the second cuff comes between 30 and 100 milliseconds later, and has no influence on it (Fig. 8.25). However, as soon as continuous flow occurs, the time delay virtually disappears, being reduced to about 1 millisecond. Both puffs occur at the same time, and the air flow from the lower cuff diverts the air flow from the upper cuff away from the sensor, and the alternating signal ceases. This rapid change of signal is used to lock another meter to give diastolic pressure. It is of interest, that the diastolic pressure recorded by this method usually lies between Phase IV and Phase V of the Korotkov sounds, and is more nearly related to Phase V.

The triple cuff method is the basis of most viable indirect systems for the regular monitoring of blood pressure. It is extremely expensive, and it is reasonable to doubt whether anything, except historical habit, can justify it.

APPENDIX

Undamped natural frequency

$$(f_0) \propto \frac{1}{2\pi} \sqrt{\frac{S}{M}} \tag{1}$$

Stiffness of diaphragm is usually quoted as volume displacement (E, in $mm^3/100\ mmHg$) which is the reciprocal of stiffness.

Therefore,

$$f_0 \propto \frac{1}{2\pi} \sqrt{\frac{1}{M \times E}} \tag{2}$$

M is the combined mass of diaphragm and liquid in transducer/catheter system. The mass of the diaphragm is small and can be ignored.

However, M in the above equation is not synonymous with the true mass, since in this system different components of the mass move with different velocities, and therefore take and give up different amounts of kinetic energy. Now,

$$\text{kinetic energy} = \text{mv}^2$$

and a doubling of the velocity would involve a 4-fold change in kinetic energy. Therefore, all components of the mass must be equalised as far as energy content is concerned by multiplying by the square of the velocity. Since equal volumes move in all parts of the system (saline is assumed to be incompressible), the differing velocities must vary inversely with the area of the part, i.e. when the cross-sectional area is halved, a given volume of fluid will have to traverse it with doubled velocity. Combining these two corrections means that the actual mass of any part of the system must be divided by the square of the cross-sectional area of that part.

Taking the mass term alone this means

$$\text{true mass} = l \times \pi \times r^2 \times \rho$$

where l and r are the length and radius of the part, and ρ (pronounced 'row') is the density of saline ($\simeq 1$ and can be ignored)

$$\text{'equivalent mass'} = \frac{\text{true mass}}{\text{area squared}} = \frac{l \times \pi r^2}{\pi r^2 \times \pi r^2} = \frac{l}{\pi r^2}$$

Substituting for M in (2)

$$f_0 \propto \frac{1}{2\pi} \sqrt{\frac{\pi r^2}{l \times E}}$$

Consider a transducer 2 cm diameter and 1 cm long, and catheter 2 mm diameter and 1 metre long:

true mass within transducer $1 \times 1^2 \pi \rho = 1\pi\rho$ grammes

true mass within catheter $= 100 \times 0 \cdot 1^2 \pi\rho = 1\pi\rho$ grammes 'equivalent' mass within transducer $\equiv \dfrac{1 \times 1^2 \times \pi}{(1^2 \times \pi) \times (1^2 \times \pi)}$

$$\equiv \frac{1}{1^2 \times \pi} \equiv \frac{1}{\pi}$$

'equivalent' mass in catheter $\equiv \dfrac{100 \times 0{\cdot}1^2 \times \pi}{(0{\cdot}1^2 \times \pi) \times (0{\cdot}1^2 \times \pi)}$

$$\equiv \frac{100}{0{\cdot}01\pi} \equiv \frac{10,000}{\pi}$$

i.e. the true mass is the same in the catheter and transducer, but the equivalent mass in the catheter, in terms of energy requirements, is 10,000 times greater than the mass in the transducer, and is therefore the only effective mass worth considering.

REFERENCES

AMERICAN HEART ASSOCIATION (1967). Recommendations for human blood pressure sphygmomanometry. Circulation **3**, 6–9, 86.

BARRY C.T. (1950) Oscillometry during anaesthesia. *Anaesthesia*, **5**, 26.

CRUL J.F. (1962) Measurement of arterial pressure. *Acta anaesthesiologica Scandinavica*, Suppl. **XI**, 135.

DEBRUNNER F. & BÜHLER F. (1969). 'Normal central venous pressure', significance of reference point and normal range. *British Medical Journal*, **3**, 148.

DE DOBBELEER G.D.P. (1963) Measurement of the systolic and diastolic blood pressure by means of phase shift. Proceedings of the 5th International Conference of Medical Electronics, Liège. Quoted in Gruen W. (1968).

FINK B.R. (1963) Pneumatic monitor for arterial blood pressure. *Anesthesiology*, **24**, 872.

GRUEN W. (1968) An assessment of present automated methods of indirect blood pressure measurements. *Annals of the New York Academy of Sciences*, **147**, Art 3, 109.

IRVINE R.O. (1968) The influence of arm girth and cuff size on the measurement of blood pressure. *New Zealand Medical Journal*, **67**, 279.

SYKES M.K. (1963) Venous pressure as a clinical indication of adequacy of transfusion. *Annals of the Royal College of Surgeons of England*, **33**, 185.

WINSOR T. & BURCH, G.E. (1945) The phlebostatic axis and phlebostatic level, reference levels for venous pressure measurements in man. *Proceedings of the Society for Experimental Biology and Medicine*, **58**, 165.

ZORAB J.S.M. (1969) Continuous display of the arterial pressure. A simple manometric technique. *Anaesthesia*, **24**, 431.

9

Measurement of Flow

Measurements of flow are standardised by collecting a measured quantity of liquid or gas in a known time. From this the mean flow rate can be calculated. The accuracy of this type of measurement depends on the accuracy with which the volume and time can be measured. Usually this is no problem. However, if gas volume is being measured (e.g. by spirometer) errors sometimes arise because of the inertia of the collecting apparatus or changes in temperature of the gas. Spirometers which can be used for calibrating flowmeters are described in Chapter 10.

More refined techniques are required when instantaneous flow rate has to be determined. The simplest techniques usually involve the measurement of the pressure drop across a fixed resistance. However, the imposition of a resistance to flow may in itself alter flow rate, so that more complicated techniques have been developed, particularly for measurement of blood flow. Many of the techniques which are applicable to the direct measurement of flow in blood vessels cannot be used to measure gaseous flow so the measurement of gaseous and liquid flow rates will be discussed separately.

MEASUREMENT OF GASEOUS FLOW

Pressure drop across a resistance
Flowmeters utilising this principle are of two types. In one, the *variable orifice* flowmeter, there is a constant pressure difference across an orifice or annular space, the cross-sectional area of the latter varying with the flow rate of the gas. In the other type, the *fixed orifice* flowmeter, the cross-sectional area of the orifice is maintained constant and, as a consequence, the pressure drop across the orifice varies with the gas flow rate.

Variable orifice flowmeters

Rotameter. This type of flowmeter has now displaced most of the other types of flowmeter previously used in anaesthesia. Although it was patented in Aachen in 1908 and first used in anaesthesia in 1910, it was not fitted to the Boyle's machine until 1937.

A rotameter consists of a vertical glass tube inside which rotates a light metal alloy bobbin. When the fine-adjustment valve (Fig. 9.1) at the bottom of the rotameter is opened the

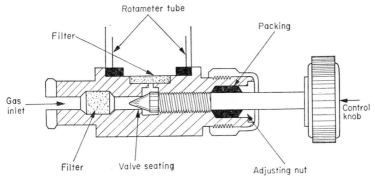

FIG. 9.1. Fine-adjustment valve to control gas flow into rotameter tube.

bobbin is forced up the tube. The inside of the tube is cone-shaped, so that the cross-sectional area of the annular space around the bobbin is greater at the top end of the tube than it is at the bottom. The height at which the bobbin settles is therefore determined by the weight of the bobbin and the pressure drop created by the flow of gas through the annular space around the bobbin. Since the weight of the bobbin is constant, the bobbin will rise until the cross-sectional area of the annular space yields a pressure drop which exactly opposes the downward pressure resulting from the weight of the bobbin. The pressure drop therefore remains constant throughout the range of flows for which the tube is designed, and the bobbin floats freely in the stream of gas. Friction between the bobbin and tube wall

5

is avoided by adding vanes to the bobbin so that it rotates in the stream of gas, and additional stability at low flow rates is achieved by modifying the shape of the bobbin (Fig. 9.2).

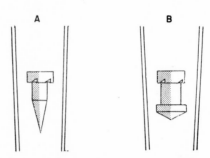

FIG. 9.2. Rotameter tubes showing (left) original shaped bobbin and (right) bobbin modified to increase stability at low flow rates.

Each rotameter has to be calibrated for a specific gas. The reason for this becomes apparent when the physical principles

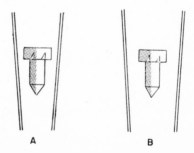

FIG. 9.3. Physical principles underlying measurement of flow by rotameter. Left: at the bottom of the tube the length of the annular space is greater than the distance between tube and bobbin. Right: at the top of the tube the annular space approximates to an orifice.

are considered (Fig. 9.3). At the bottom of the rotameter the length of the bobbin is much greater than the distance between the bobbin and glass. The channel therefore approximates to a tube and, providing flow is laminar, viscosity is an important determinant of pressure drop:

$$\text{pressure difference} \propto \frac{\text{viscosity} \times \text{length} \times \text{flow rate}}{(\text{radius})^4}$$

As the bobbin rises, the distance between bobbin and tube increases, so that the space around the bobbin approximates

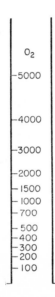

Fɪɢ. 9.4. A linear scale on rotameter.

more to an orifice than to a tube. For flow through an orifice the density becomes an important factor (the pressure drop is directly proportional to the density of the gas and to the square of the velocity). Since the transition from a tubular space to an orifice is not clearly defined, and since a certain amount of turbulence must occur even at low flow rates, it is apparent that each rotameter must be calibrated specifically for one gas. Furthermore, since viscosity and density vary with temperature, the calibration must be carried out at the appropriate temperature. If these precautions are observed, and the rotameter is mounted vertically and kept clean, the reading (taken from the top of the bobbin) should be accurate to within ±2 per cent of the true value.

Further complexities in calibration have resulted from the introduction of rotameters in which portions of the scale are expanded so that increased accuracy of reading is available over

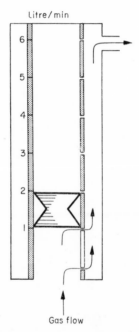

FIG. 9.5. Coxeter flowmeter.

specific ranges of flow. This feature is made possible by varying the taper of the cone in different parts of the tube. However, if the scale is read carelessly or the marking is not clear, serious errors can result from incorrect gas flow settings. The anaesthetist should therefore always check the scale to observe where the deviations from linearity occur, before using the machine (Fig. 9.4).

Coxeter flowmeter. This flowmeter was fitted to the Boyle's machine from about 1933 to 1937. The bobbin was machined to provide a close fit with a glass tube of uniform bore (Fig. 9.5). When gas entered the tube from below the bobbin was displaced upwards until gas started to escape through one of the holes in the side of the tube. The height of the bobbin was determined by the number of holes which had to be exposed to the gas flow before the pressure drop equalled the downward pressure exerted by the bobbin. Since the number of holes was somewhat limited,

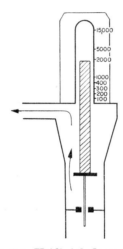

FIG. 9.6. Heidbrink flowmeter.

the bobbin rose in a series of steps as gas flow was increased, the actual flow rate being indicated by the reading on the scale opposite the top of the bobbin. The bobbin tended to stick and dirt sometimes partially occluded the holes, so that the meter was not very accurate.

Heidbrink flowmeter. This meter has been widely used in the United States. Again, the position of the plunger in the conical tube depends on the balance between the downward pressure exerted by the plunger and the pressure drop across the annular orifice. The scale is non-linear, to facilitate its use in closed-circuit anaesthesia (Fig. 9.6).

Inclined tube flowmeter. The conical glass tube was mounted at an angle to the horizontal and a ball was used to indicate flow.

In the original design of Ewing a single ball was used (Fig. 9.7). This, however, tended to oscillate: the use of two balls on the flowmeters fitted to the Connell Stratosphere machine ensured stability. The reading was taken from the point of contact of the balls.

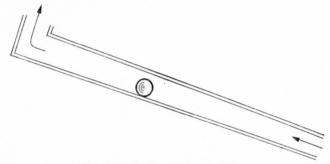

FIG. 9.7. Inclined tube flowmeter.

Variable-pressure flowmeters

Water-depression flowmeter. This type of flowmeter was widely used in the United States on Foregger anaesthetic machines. There were two basic designs (Fig. 9.8). In one the gas was

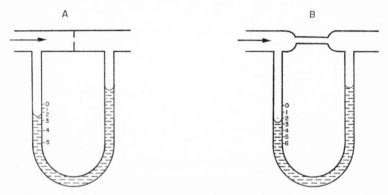

FIG. 9.8. Water-depression flowmeters. (A) Orifice type with alinear scale. (B) Laminar flow type with linear scale.

caused to flow through an orifice and the pressure drop across the orifice was measured with a water manometer. Since the pressure drop across an orifice is proportional to the square of the flow rate, the scale was alinear, being crowded at the lower readings and expanded at the higher readings. This was obviously undesirable for anaesthesia, and so parallel-sided tubes were substituted for the orifice. This ensured that flow was laminar, and consequently the pressure drop was proportional to flow rate: a linear scale could therefore be obtained. It was, however, necessary to provide a number of flowmeters in parallel to obtain accuracy over a wide range of flow rates, and there was always the danger of blowing water into the patient circuit when the cylinders were suddenly opened.

Bourdon gauge flowmeter. In this instrument a Bourdon gauge is used to sense the pressure drop across an orifice (Fig. 9.9). The meter is rugged, not affected by changes in position, and therefore

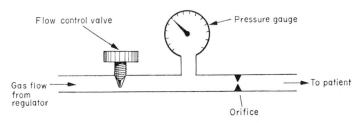

FIG. 9.9. Bourdon gauge flowmeter.

useful for metering the flow from cylinders of gases which are used when transporting patients from one place to another. It is, however, affected by back pressure (see p. 129). In some types of meter an aneroid system is used instead of the Bourdon gauge to detect the pressure difference.

Pneumotachograph. In order to maintain laminar flow at the high flow rates encountered during respiration, the pneumotachograph employs a number of parallel-sided tubes as the resistance to gas flow. In the Fleisch head the tubes are formed by rolling a strip of corrugated foil into a cylinder (Fig. 9.10). A number of holes are situated around the tube at each end of the resistance. These lead into annular chambers which are connected to the pressure manometer by flexible tubes. The pressure drop across this resistance is small (0–10 mm H_2O at flows up to 250 litres/min depending on the particular head used) and a sensitive differential pressure transducer is therefore required to measure it. The Lilley type of pneumotachograph head uses a heated gauze as the resistance and also requires a sensitive transducer to measure the pressure difference.

The signal from a pneumotachograph head is rarely completely linearly related to flow, but by suitable design it is usually

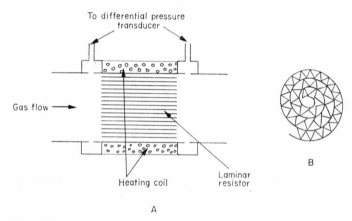

FIG. 9.10. Pneumotachograph. A. longitudinal section. B. Transverse section showing corrugated foil wound into a spiral.

possible to use such an instrument within a known range of flows to obtain an accuracy of about ± 5 per cent. Calibration depends on the viscosity of the gas passing across the resistance, and this is in turn dependent on temperature and the composition of the gas mixture (Hobbs 1967). Condensation of water vapour on the resistance also affects the calibration but can be minimised by heating the resistance with an electric heating element.

Two other types of variable-pressure flowmeter must be mentioned, although they have not been widely used clinically.

Venturi tube flowmeter. When gas passes through a narrowed portion of tube it accelerates. Some potential energy is thus converted to kinetic energy and the pressure recorded from a side arm in the constricted part of the tube is less than the pressure in the wider part of the tube (Fig. 9.11). Because the pressure difference is roughly proportional to the square of the flow rate, the scale is non-linear, sensitivity being least at low flow rates. Furthermore, the instrument is very sensitive to changes in the density of the gas.

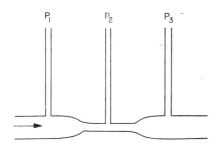

FIG. 9.11. Venturi tube flowmeter. Pressure in $P_1 > P_2$. P_3 is measured if flow is reversed.

Pitot tube flowmeter. This again utilises the difference between the amount of potential and kinetic energy possessed by the gas. The potential energy is proportional to its pressure, and the kinetic energy is proportional to its velocity. In the pitot tube

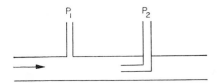

FIG. 9.12. Pitot tube flowmeter.

flowmeter (Fig. 9.12) the kinetic energy is sensed by the difference in pressure between a tube facing into the stream of gas and a tube measuring the lateral pressure exerted by the gas. This pressure difference is proportional to the square of flow rate, so that the scale is again non-linear. Furthermore the range of flow which can be accommodated by any particular instrument is somewhat limited.

5*

Water-sight flowmeter. This type of flowmeter was used in the earlier models of the Boyle's machine (Fig. 9.13). Since the pressure drop and size of orifice both varied it fell into neither of the above classifications. The gas escaped through one or more holes bored in the side of a tube dipping under water. The pressure drop across the hole was balanced by the hydrostatic pressure of the external water column. If flow rate was increased the pressure drop across the hole was increased and the water

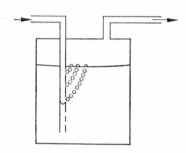

Fig. 9.13. Water-sight flowmeter.

in the flowmeter tube was forced down until the gas could escape through a lower hole. Observation of the lowest hole through which the gas was bubbling yielded a measure of flow rate. The height of water in the reservoir had to be kept constant and high flows of gas could not be used since the resultant excessive bubbling prevented proper observation of the tubes.

Effect of pressure on flowmeters

The pressure within a flowmeter may be altered by an alteration in ambient pressure or by an alteration in the resistance to outflow. The effects of alterations in ambient pressure are seen at altitude or when the flowmeter is used in a hyperbaric chamber. Alterations in outflow resistance are more commonly encountered and may be caused by the attachment of anaesthetic vaporizers, nebulisers or gas-driven ventilators (e.g. the Manley).

Under hyperbaric conditions the density of the gas is increased so that at a given flow rate a larger orifice will be necessary to maintain the same pressure difference. In other words a rota-meter will read high in a pressure chamber. McDowall (1964) has found that the actual flow (F_A) is given by the equation:

$$F_A = F_I \times \sqrt{\frac{\rho_0}{\rho_1}}$$

where F_I is the indicated flow under hyperbaric conditions whilst ρ_0 and ρ_1 are the densities of the gas at atmospheric and hyperbaric pressures respectively. Thus, if pressure is increased to two atmospheres absolute, density is doubled and

$$\sqrt{\frac{\rho_0}{\rho_1}} = \sqrt{\tfrac{1}{2}}$$

so that F_A is 71 per cent of F_I. It should be noted that F_A is the volume flow rate which is measured under the hyperbaric conditions existing in the chamber. Similar reasoning indicates that with a constant orifice meter (e.g. Bourdon gauge meter) the pressure difference for a given flow rate will be greater under hyperbaric conditions, so that this too will read high.

When a back pressure is exerted on the outlet from a rotameter by a nebuliser or ventilator the bobbin falls. For all practical purposes the flow which is now indicated is correct, although the actual reduction in flow is slightly greater than that indicated on the flowmeter. The flow control must therefore be set to indicate slightly more than the desired flow after the ventilator has been attached. The effect is substantially the same for both oxygen and nitrous oxide. Back pressure also causes a constant orifice meter to read high. Indeed, with a Bourdon gauge flow-meter complete occlusion of the outlet tube causes the pressure in the tube to build up until it equals the outlet pressure set on the reducing valve. The meter will therefore indicate maximum flow when flow is zero.

The problems introduced by back pressure on rotameters can be easily overcome by placing the fine-adjustment flow control valve on the outlet side of the rotameter instead of the inlet side. The gas in the tube is thus constantly pressurised to regulator-outlet pressure, and back pressure effects are minimised. Special precautions have to be taken to prevent leaks from the rotameter, and the flowmeter must be calibrated under the correct pressure conditions, but such *pressure-compensated* flowmeters are now being widely adopted for general use.

Other sources of inaccuracy in flowmeters

One of the main sources of inaccuracy is that there is a leak in the circuit between the flowmeter and patient. This may lead to errors in the concentration of gas delivered (Eger & Epstein 1964). Another source of error is sticking of the rotameter due to the presence of dirt or to the accumulation of a static charge (Hagelsten & Larsen 1965).

Other devices for measuring gas flow

Thermistor flowmeter. This consists of a small thermistor mounted in a tube. The change in temperature between inspired and expired air produces cyclical changes in temperature, which can be displayed on a meter. Whilst this device is useful as a qualitative monitor of respiration, quantification is almost impossible. However, if the temperature and composition of the flowing gas is constant, the cooling effect on a heated wire or heated thermistor can be used to measure flowrate.

Ultrasonic flowmeter. A gas flowmeter working on this principle has just been introduced as part of a system for respiratory function testing. The apparatus utilises the difference in velocity of transmission of ultrasound from two crystals placed diagonally across a flowing gas stream. The velocity is increased when the gas flows in the direction of the sound and is decreased when gas flows in the opposite direction. It is claimed that the signal is little affected by moisture or normal changes in composition of respired gas and that the measurement can be made without introducing any resistance into the system.

The peak flowmeter

The peak expiratory flow rate which can be achieved by normal adults often exceeds 500 litres/min. Peak flow can be measured by a pneumotachograph, but a more useful clinical instrument is the peak flowmeter (Wright and McKerrow 1959). This is basically a variable-area orifice meter and is capable of measuring flows up to 1000 litre/min, with the imposition of only a small resistance to gas flow.

The meter consists of a metal cylinder about 12 cm in diameter and 4 cm deep. A mouthpiece is attached to one side of the cylinder and a fixed partition deflects the expired air onto a movable vane (Fig. 9.14). The vane fits the inside of the cylinder

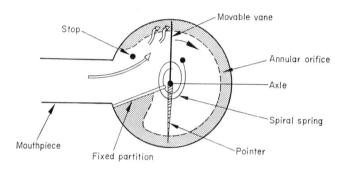

FIG. 9.14. Peak expiratory flowmeter.

closely and is free to rotate around a central axle. The air flow forces the vane to rotate against the pressure exerted by a spiral spring and the movement of the vane then opens up an annular orifice which permits the air to escape to the outside. As the pressure exerted by the spiral spring only increases minimally as the vane rotates, the position adopted by the vane depends primarily on the flow rate and on the area of the annular orifice which must be exposed to the air flow to maintain a constant pressure difference. The vane is very light and hence rapidly attains a maximum position in response to the peak expiratory flow. It is then retained in this position by a ratchet, which can be released after the reading has been taken. The reading is obtained from a pointer which is attached at an angle of 180° to the vane, and so balances it. The meter tends to under-read slightly when compared with the peak expiratory flow rate recorded by a pneumotachograph, but there is a consistent relation between the two measurements.

Fast spirometers. Wet or dry spirometers can be used to record flow rate over limited periods of time. If a wet spirometer (Fig. 10.1) is used it must conform to a specification which ensures that it will adequately follow rapid changes in flow rate (Bernstein, D'Silva & Mendel 1952). The unmodified Benedict–Roth type of spirometer is therefore not suitable for this purpose. Dry spirometers (such as the Vitalograph) are now highly developed and more convenient than the wet variety. In the Vitalograph the movement of a wedged-shaped bellows is recorded on a chart which runs for 6 seconds. The capacity of the bellows is 6 litres and the accuracy of recording within ±1 per cent. To conserve chart space it is arranged that the chart only begins to move when the patient starts to breathe out. Flow rate can be computed from the slope of the resulting trace.

DIRECT METHODS FOR MEASURING LIQUID FLOW

Similar methods of measurement to those described in the previous section can also be applied to the measurement of liquid flow. However, the much greater density and viscosity of fluid necessitates a number of modifications to the apparatus. Many of these methods are used in industry and some have been adapted to the measurement of flow in the heart–lung and artificial kidney machines.

Measurement of mean flow

A number of relatively simple instruments have been used in physiological research to measure mean flow. The simplest method is to divert the flow into a graduated vessel for a known time. To prevent alterations in the circulation due to loss of blood the Ludwig stromuhr can be utilised (Fig. 9.15).

Rotameters have found a wide application in industry and medicine. The basic principle is similar to the gas rotameter, but the movement of the bobbin is sensed by recording the change in inductance in a coil when a soft-iron core attached to the rotameter rises within the coil (Fig. 9.16). By careful design the effect of viscosity changes in the blood can be minimised so that calibration does not change appreciably with changing haematocrit.

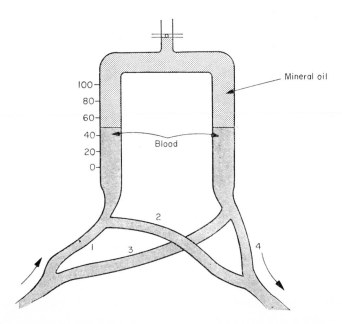

FIG. 9.15. Ludwig stromuhr. Blood normally flows in the direction shown by arrows. When tubes 2 and 3 are clamped blood flows into one chamber and out of the other. By using a stop watch it is possible to calculate the flow rate. On the next occasion tubes 1 and 4 are clamped to reverse the flow.

Another instrument utilising a rotating vane is the Potter electroturbinometer. In this instrument the vane is built around a permanent magnet and fixed so that it can rotate in a tube which is inserted between the cut ends of a blood vessel. The speed of rotation of the rotor is sensed by a pick-up coil situated in the wall of the instrument. This instrument is remarkably stable and is capable of an accuracy of ±5 per cent. However, the resistance to flow is greater than with a good rotameter and it ceases to rotate at very low flows.

Heat-dissipation methods have also proved popular. The thermostromuhr is an example of an instrument which has been widely used. In one of the more recent modifications two thermistors are placed in close apposition to the blood vessel. The thermistors are separated by a heating coil and it is arranged that their electrical outputs oppose each other. When the heating

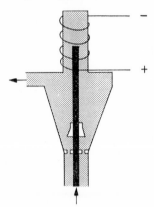

FIG. 9.16. Liquid rotameter.

coil is switched on the downstream thermistor will record a higher temperature than the upstream thermistor. The difference in temperature between the two thermistors is inversely related to blood flow. This instrument is reasonably accurate if flow is non-pulsatile, but may become very inaccurate when pulsatile flow is present.

Other heat-dissipation methods have been used. One of the simplest was a length of resistance wire passed down the length of the blood vessel. An electrical current was passed down the wire to heat it, and the loss of heat, which was proportional to blood flow, was detected by measuring the change in resistance of the wire. A similar catheter tip flowmeter utilising thermistors has been used more recently. However the increasing availability of methods for measuring pulsatile flow has rendered most of the above methods obsolete.

Measurement of oscillatory flow

Pressure gradient method. This method is technically easy to perform, but the mathematical treatment is so complex that it has not so far been employed clinically. It will be recalled that Poiseuille's formula (p. 121) relates the flow through a tube to the dimensions of the tube, the nature of the liquid, and the pressure difference applied to it. An unbranched segment of a vessel can be regarded as a tube, and if its diameter can be ascertained, then the flow within it can be calculated from the pressure gradient across a length of the tube. However, as the flow is oscillatory and has a complex waveform, the pressure difference is constantly changing. It is therefore necessary to record the instantaneous values of pressure between two points in the vessel. These can be measured by a double lumen catheter and a differential transducer. The system must fulfil stringent criteria for frequency response and damping, for reasons outlined in the section on intra-arterial blood pressure measurement (Chapter 8). The first step in the analysis is to partition the wave into its component sine waves by a Fourier analysis. Poiseuille's equation has then to be solved for many small increments for each significant harmonic and summated. An on-line computer would no doubt perform this analysis rapidly enough to enable the results to be available in a reasonable time, but even if this were possible, the calculation would still require a knowledge of the diameter of the vessel. It is not clear to what extent the pulsatile changes associated with each beat would affect a result based, for example, on a radiographic measurement. It is clearly a long step before this method could find routine application.

Electromagnetic blood flowmeters. There are many varieties of this instrument but all depend on the principle that if blood or other electrolyte flows at right-angles to a magnetic field then an e.m.f. will be induced in a plane mutually at right angles to the magnetic field and to the direction of fluid flow (Fig. 9.17). The induced voltage is proportional to the average cross-sectional velocity at any moment and, since the flowmeter wraps round the blood vessel and maintains a constant vessel diameter, the velocity signal can be read in terms of volume flow. To prevent drift due to polarization of the electrodes the coils used to produce the magnetic field are energised with a square or sine wave current of between 50 and 400 Hz. The changing magnetic field also induces a back-e.m.f. which is 90° out of phase with the induced voltage, but this can be eliminated by a gating system after amplification. Unfortunately, this method of flow measurement can only be used when a vessel is exposed and tightly held within the probe head, and zero flow can be assured

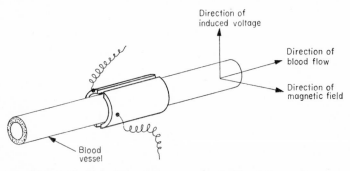

Direction of
induced voltage

Direction of
blood flow

Direction of
magnetic field

Blood
vessel

FIG. 9.17. Principle of electromagnetic blood flowmeter.

for calibration purposes. The latter condition is often difficult to achieve but is an essential requirement, since baseline drift is one of the chief sources of inaccuracy.

A more recent development of this technique utilises a coil placed in the tip of a cardiac catheter. This measures the velocity of flow at the tip of the catheter. Since the axial flow in a blood vessel is greater than the flow at the periphery, the probe is somewhat position-sensitive. In large vessels such as the aorta the velocity profile is much flatter than in small vessels, so that the positional error is not great. However, flow probes all suffer from the disadvantage that the vessel diameter must be determined by radiographic techniques before volume flow can be calculated. An alternative method for determining volume flow in the aorta is to calibrate the flow probe against direct determinations of cardiac output.

Ultrasonic blood flowmeters. This type of flowmeter has been developed intensively over the past ten years. A probe surrounds the vessel and a small piezo-electric crystal is mounted in the wall of each half of the probe. One crystal transmits sound diagonally across the vessel and the other receives it. The direction of transmission of sound between the crystals is alternated several hundred times a second, the sound frequency varying in different instruments from 100 kHz to 8 MHz. Since sound waves travel more rapidly downstream than upstream, the difference between the two velocities may be used to measure blood flow. Although the principle is easy to comprehend, its practical fulfilment has been delayed owing to the enormous technical difficulties in detecting the very small differences in the velocity of sound between the two directions in which it is propagated.

Two methods of detecting this difference are used. One method depends on the measurement of the phase shift of the sound picked up by the receiver. In the other type of instrument the sound waves are emitted in very short pulses with an interval between each pulse. The pulses alternate in direction and the instrument measures the time interval between the emission and reception of the pulse in each direction.

Ultrasonic flowmeters also have the disadvantage that they measure the *velocity* of flow and not the *volume* of flow. However, the latter can be calculated if the cross-sectional area of the vessel and the velocity profile are known. These instruments have already proved useful as an investigative tool. A catheter-tip ultrasonic probe has also been recently introduced. Like other catheter probes it measures velocity at one point in the vessel and so is affected by the velocity profile existing within the vessel. A commercial instrument utilising the ultrasonic principle has recently been used for detecting air emboli during anaesthesia (Edmonds-Seal & Maroon 1969). It is extremely sensitive and can detect volumes of air down to 0·25 ml.

Bristle flowmeters. This type of flowmeter is now obsolete but was used extensively for the investigation of venous return. A bristle was inserted into the blood stream at right-angles to the direction of flow. Movement of this bristle was sensed by attaching it to the anode pin of a special transducer vacuum valve. The output voltage from this valve was used to drive a recorder.

INDIRECT METHODS FOR MEASURING LIQUID FLOW

Attempts have been made to measure cardiac output by taking multiple radiographs of the heart, by examination of the arterial pulse contour and by studying the oscillations induced in the body by the heart beat (ballisto-cardiography). However, none of these methods maintained sufficient accuracy throughout the whole of the physiological range of cardiac output, so they will not be described further.

INDICATOR TECHNIQUES FOR MEASURING LIQUID FLOW: GENERAL PRINCIPLES

The Fick principle

The Fick principle was enunciated in 1870 and has since formed the basis of many techniques for measuring liquid flow. The principle applies to any flowing stream of liquid when a substance either enters or leaves the stream. The principle states that the flow of liquid in a given period of time is equal to the amount of substance entering or leaving the stream in the same period of time, divided by the difference between the concentrations of the substance before and after the point of entry or exit (Fig. 9.18).

When measuring cardiac output the uptake of oxygen or elimination of carbon dioxide from the blood is utilised. If the arterio-venous content difference is known then the flow can be calculated from the O_2 or CO_2 exchange in the lung. For example, if the arterio-venous O_2 difference is 5 vols per cent, then 5 ml of O_2 must be exchanged for every 100 ml of blood flowing through the lungs. If the oxygen consumption is 300 ml/min then the cardiac output must be

$$\frac{300}{5} \times 100 \text{ ml} = 6000 \text{ ml} = 6 \text{ litres/min}$$

i.e.

cardiac output (litres/min)

$$= \frac{O_2 \text{ consumption (ml/min)}}{\text{arterio-venous } O_2 \text{ content difference (ml/litre)}}$$

Similar calculations can be applied to CO_2. One of the main problems in this *direct Fick* method is the difficulty of obtaining a sample of mixed venous blood. Mixed venous P_{CO_2} (but not

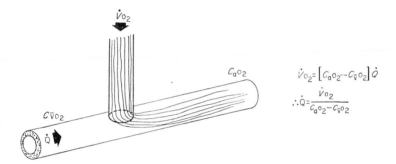

FIG. 9.18. Fick principle.

P_{O_2}) can be estimated by the rebreathing technique (page 193) and CO_2 content calculated from the CO_2 dissociation curve, but the accuracy of such an *indirect Fick method* is inadequate for most clinical work. Furthermore, large errors result from the use of CO_2 as an indicator gas if changes in alveolar and arterial P_{CO_2} occur during the course of the measurements. The Fick technique can only be applied in steady-state conditions, the limiting factor being the accuracy of measurement of O_2 consumption or CO_2 output (usually ± 10 per cent). Despite the technical difficulties and other objections to the method (Visscher & Johnson 1953) this still remains the standard by which other methods are judged.

The Fick principle is also used indirectly in methods based on the absorption of a foreign gas by the blood during its passage through the lungs. If the solubility of the gas in blood is known and its uptake is measured, blood flow can be calculated. This technique has been chiefly used with acetylene and nitrous oxide. Other indicator techniques utilise the Fick principle. Two are in common use.

Constant-infusion indicator dilution. A substance is injected into one part of the circulation at a constant rate and its concentration is then sampled elsewhere. From the dilution of the injected solution it is possible to calculate flow rate, providing that recirculation does not occur. This limits the use of the technique to situations where the injected substance is destroyed rapidly. The general formula then simplifies to

$$\text{cardiac output} = \frac{\text{rate of infusion of indicator}}{\text{concentration of indicator in blood}}$$

Various modifications of this technique are possible to suit various applications. Some of these are discussed more fully later in this chapter.

Single-injection indicator dilution. In this technique an indicator is injected as a 'slug' into the vena cava, the right heart or, preferably, the pulmonary artery. The concentration of the indicator is then sampled continuously from the systemic side of the circulation, measured spectrophotometrically and plotted against time. The flow is worked out in the following manner. Suppose that 5 mg of indicator was injected, that the duration of the curve was 30 seconds, and that the mean concentration of the indicator was 2 mg/litre (the latter is calculated from the area under the curve divided by the duration of the curve.) Then the 5 mg of indicator must have been diluted by $\frac{5}{2} = 2 \cdot 5$ litres of blood during the 30 seconds. Hence, the cardiac output must have been $\frac{60}{30} \times 2 \cdot 5 = 5$ litres/min.

The general formula is:

$$\text{cardiac output}$$
$$= \frac{60 \times \text{indicator dose (in mg)}}{\text{average concentration} \times \text{time (in secs)}} \text{ in litres/min}$$

One of the problems with this method is that recirculation of indicator occurs before the downslope of the curve is completed (Fig. 9.19a). A number of techniques have been proposed to overcome this difficulty, but the most commonly used method utilises the exponential character of the downslope. If such a

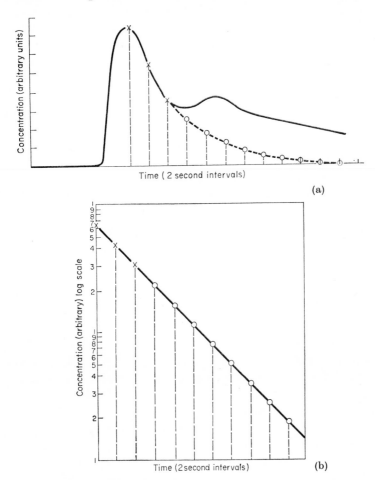

FIG. 9.19. Single-dose dye dilution curve (a) and replot on semi-logarithmic paper (b). **X** = points used to plot exponential. o = points used to plot the tail of the curve.

curve is replotted on a semi-logarithmic scale a straight line results (Fig. 9.19b). By utilising points from the top portion of the recorded dye curve the slope of the semi-logarithmic plot is established. Points from the lower portion of this slope are then replotted back onto the original curve to define the tail of the curve which would have been recorded if recirculation had not occurred (Fig. 9.19a). The area may then be measured by counting squares, weighing the paper enclosed by the curve or planimetry.* Other methods of calculating the area of the curve have been devised but all involve a variable degree of approximation. Cardiac output computers have also been devised: these essentially perform the same steps as outlined above.

A number of indicators have been used for this technique. Of the dyes used indocyanine green (Cardio-green or Fox-green) has proved most popular. It is non-toxic, it does not interfere with the colorimetric estimation of oxygen saturation, and it has a relatively short half-life, so that repeated measurements can be made. Dye curves have also been inscribed using radioactive tracers, saline (using an electrical conductivity detector) and cold saline (using a thermal detector).

Clearance techniques

Another method which is used particularly for the measurement of tissue blood flow utilises the measurement of the clearance of a radioactive tracer from the tissue. For example ^{24}Na or ^{133}Xe may be injected into a muscle and the rate of washout followed with a scintillation counter. Similarly, the rate of clearance of ^{133}Xe from the alveoli can provide a measure of regional pulmonary blood flow. These techniques are discussed in more detail later in this chapter.

Plethysmography

Limb plethysmography is carried out by measuring the increase in volume of a limb when the venous outflow is abolished by a cuff. The rate of rise of limb volume over the first few seconds of venous occlusion then corresponds to the rate of blood flow

---

* A planimeter is an instrument which mechanically integrates the area under the curve. In operation, one end of the instrument is fixed while the pointer on the other end is traced around the curve and baseline. The area is then read from a dial.

into the limb. Leaks between limb and box are prevented by rubber sleeves. The water-filled plethysmograph is maintained close to skin-temperature by a thermostat and heater. The increase in volume of the limb is then recorded by measuring the displacement of water or air from the box or by recording the change in pressure in an air-filled system.

A simplified form of plethysmograph described by Whitney (1953) is based on the demonstration that the change in limb girth bears a direct relation to the change in limb volume. This

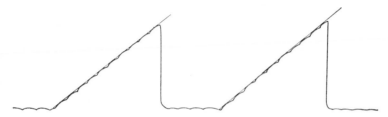

Fig. 9.20. Limb plethysmography. Recorded changes in limb volume following two occlusions of 10 seconds each.

change in girth is recorded with a mercury-in-rubber strain gauge which surrounds the limb. When the rubber tube containing the mercury is stretched it becomes narrower. The electrical resistance of the column of mercury therefore increases. This change in resistance can be detected by a Wheatstone bridge circuit and then amplified and recorded (Fig. 9.20).

The change in limb volume can also be recorded by measuring the change of electrical impedance of the limb.

RADIOISOTOPE TECHNIQUES FOR MEASURING LIQUID FLOW

Any investigation which can be performed using a dye, can usually be performed with equal simplicity using a radioactive isotope. It is thus possible to employ radioactive isotopes in a number of methods for measuring cardiac output, pulmonary blood flow, and flow through the various tissues and vessels. However, ability to detect radioactive emissions directly without recourse to samples extends the potential scope enormously. There is a vast literature on blood flow measurements in various organs, and anyone contemplating entering the field will find many useful references in Sevelius (1965), as well as a full exposition on the interpretation of data. Considerable further developments have taken place during the last few years; whilst there is very little direct application to clinical anaesthesia, there are research applications appearing in the literature, and a brief outline of their principles is therefore included. As with other indicator techniques, flow measurements fall into three basic categories; indicator dilution methods, those involving constant injection, and clearance methods.

Indicator dilution methods
It is possible to replace a dye by a radioactive isotope, and to replace a densitometer cuvette by a well counter containing a coil through which blood flows, and so to plot a time-dilution curve as in the standard Stewart–Hamilton technique for cardiac output determination.

However, the ease with which the concentration of the indicator can be measured in the intact body, has led to determined attempts to calibrate a time-dilution curve by external counting over a large vascular volume. The basic concept is still the same as that used for the standard dye method of estimating cardiac output discussed earlier. The formula is

$$\text{cardiac output} = \frac{E}{A} \times \text{blood volume}$$

where A is the area under the time-activity curve and E the recording of the same volume after complete equilibration. Blood volume is calculated from the ratio of the injected activity to the equilibrium activity in a sample of blood (see page 159). It is again of fundamental importance that the equilibrium recording must be taken over the same area and focus, with the patient's position unchanged, and at the same metabolic and dynamic state of the patient. This is its greatest limitation. However, it is possible to get an acceptable correlation between the external method and the arterial sampling method if enough attention is paid to detail (Sevelius 1965). If the detector is placed precordially, two time-dilution curves are obtained, one for each side of the heart. It is also possible to use such a radio-cardiogram to obtain the coronary blood flow.

Constant injection methods

The simplest situation in which this method is used is where the entire output, be it from a vessel or from an organ, flows through a single outlet which can be sampled. A continuous injection of a known concentration of radioactive tracer is made at a uniform rate and a sample of the diluted tracer is then withdrawn from a point at which thorough mixing can be assumed. The concentration of the diluted material is measured and then the flow is calculated from the equation:

injected concentration × flow
= blood flow × diluted concentration

This formula merely restates the concept of the conservation of matter; consequently it is only applicable to organ flow measurements where there is no uptake or removal of tracer from the blood by the organ. Since this is rarely true, the method is limited to the measurement of flow in vessels. Experimentally, it has been used as a method of measuring cardiac output, with injection taking place in the vena cava and sampling taking place from the pulmonary artery. To prevent interference from recirculated isotope, ^{133}Xe dissolved in saline is used, as this is almost completely evolved in the alveolar gas during one passage through the lungs.

A variant of this principle can be used for measuring the flow of blood through an organ if the tracer is completely removed from the blood in one passage through it. An example is the measurement of effective renal plasma flow. For this, ^{131}I-labelled hippuran is given by a constant infusion pump. An external monitor over the heart indicates when the steadily rising level of radiation in the circulation changes to an equilibrium level: at this point the kidneys are removing the label from the circulation at the same rate as it is being added. If blood samples are taken at this time for assay of activity in the plasma, the renal plasma flow is the ratio of the counts being infused to the counts in the plasma, multiplied by the rate of infusion. A simple way of visualising this is to consider it again as a problem in the conservation of mass. The mass going *into* the plasma in unit time is the concentration of the tracer multiplied by the infusion rate; the mass coming *out* of the plasma is the renal arteriovenous concentration difference multiplied by the renal plasma flow. If the venous concentration is zero, only the arterial concentration is needed, and if there is no uptake in other tissues, then the arterial concentration will be the same as the venous concentration from, say, the arm.

Clearance techniques

There are two basic forms of the clearance technique: plasma clearance and tissue clearance.

Plasma clearance. If it is possible to select an indicator which is removed from the circulation by one organ only, then a semi-logarithmic plot of the blood concentration against time is a function of tissue perfusion and is a straight line. If the indicator is fully extracted from the blood in one passage through the organ of interest, then the actual flow can be calculated provided that the distribution volume of the tracer is known. This latter condition limits the usefulness of the method. To avoid this restriction, the half-time of blood clearance may be calculated if serial comparative measurements are required, or if a simple index of effective blood flow is needed. Another expression of this function is the disappearance rate constant, which may be thought of as the fraction of the total blood volume perfusing the organ. Because of the exponential nature of the clearance process, this constant is 0·693 divided by the half-time.

The technique can still be applied in principle, even if the extraction efficiency of the organ in question is not 100 per cent. If quantitative measurements are required, the outflow of blood from the organ must be assayed. If only the half-time is required, this is not necessary.

Tissue clearance. There are two main variations of technique. One variation is exemplified by the technique of measuring muscle blood flow by measuring the rate of removal of radioactive ^{24}Na-labelled NaCl which has been directly injected into the muscle. The alternative technique is to perfuse the tissue with a continuous infusion of tracer until the tissue is in a steady state, and then to monitor the rate of fall in activity in the tissue after the perfusion is stopped. Such a method is utilised in the technique of Ingvar & Lassen (1961) for the measurement of cerebral blood flow.

Blood flow through particular areas of cerebral cortex can be measured during craniotomy, using ^{85}Kr. This is a weak-emitter and is not detectable through the intact skull. A similar technique can be applied through the intact skull using external gamma-counters employing either ^{79}Kr or ^{133}Xe, but this measures flow in a whole slice of brain. The half-life of ^{79}Kr is 34 hours, and this makes it relatively less convenient than ^{133}Xe. In both open and closed skull methods the isotope is injected at a constant rate into the internal carotid artery until the radiation being detected in the cerebral cortex becomes steady. Infusion is then stopped and the washout process is recorded, the rate of blood flow being inversely proportional to the rate of fall of radioactivity. The clearance is usually expressed in terms of a half-time of clearance, that is, the time taken for the measured radioactivity to fall to half its initial value. Veall & Mallett (1966), have modified the technique so that the isotope is administered by inhalation rather than by intracarotid injection. The recorded clearance curve is proportional to the cortical perfusion rate, but to obtain absolute values it is necessary to subject the data to complex mathematical analysis.

It is an important restriction of tissue-clearance techniques that the distribution coefficient of tracer between the blood and tissue must greatly favour the blood, and that the transfer of tracer from tissue to blood should be as rapid as possible. The clearance rate is related not only to the flow rate through the tissue, but also to the rate of transfer from tissue to blood. Only when this transfer is very rapid is clearance related in a simple fashion to flow rate. If transfer is not rapid, then clearance may be almost independent of flow rate. A fuller mathematical exposition is given by Powers & Sevelius (1965).

Providing that the vessel perfusing the relevant organ can be cannulated, the inert gas clearance method can always be applied to it. It has been applied, not only for the brain, but to the coronary arteries, to muscles, skin, kidneys and liver. As yet, radioactive techniques have been little employed (apart from cerebral blood flow) to measurements of flow in various organs during anaesthesia. The complex apparatus used in external monitoring is rarely compatible with surgery, or at any rate, with surgical access. Nevertheless, there are many applications which are possible, and it is likely that this will prove to be a rapidly expanding field in the future.

Pulmonary ventilation and pulmonary blood flow

The use of radioactive gases to measure the distribution of ventilation in the lung was pioneered by Knipping and his colleagues in 1955. These workers used Geiger counters placed over different regions of the lung to measure the distribution of ^{133}Xe. Later, Dyson and his colleagues (1960) used radioactive oxygen to measure regional differences in pulmonary blood flow.

Radioactive methods used today may be divided into those employing 'very soluble' or 'poorly soluble' gases, the 'solubility' in this context referring to the ease with which these gases are absorbed into the pulmonary capillary blood. The soluble gases are oxygen and carbon dioxide. The suitable isotopes of these gases, from the point of view of their emissions, are both of very short half-life and have to be piped directly from the cyclotron to the laboratory. To measure the distribution of pulmonary blood flow the patient is seated between a number of detectors covering different regions of the chest. A breath of radioactive gas is then inhaled and the counting rates are observed while the breath is held. The rate of fall of activity during the breath-holding period is proportional to the blood flow in the area of lung being scanned by the counters.

Relatively insoluble isotopes are ^{133}Xe and ^{13}N. Since ^{13}N has to be prepared in a cyclotron, its use has been somewhat limited. and it is now ^{133}Xe which is most widely used. The latter has a half-life of 5·3 days and can be dissolved in saline under pressure. There are a number of different techniques which utilise this isotope. In one, the dissolved xenon is injected as a bolus into a catheter in the superior vena cava. When the gas reaches the pulmonary capillaries, it is evolved into the alveoli because of its low solubility. If the subject holds his breath during this period, the rate of rise of radioactivity counted over the chest provides a measure of pulmonary blood flow. In practice, the lung is scanned either with multiple stationary counters or with moving counters during this period. The shape of the tracing represents the blood flow and the volume of the lung at various points throughout the lung. To eliminate the geometrical factors, a second scan is made after the subject has rebreathed the xenon in and out of a bag. This ensures that all the alveolar gas is uniformly labelled and the scan which results shows the record which would have been obtained if all the alveoli had been evenly perfused. The difference between the first and second scans therefore represents regional differences in blood flow. Usually, however, the ordinates of the first scan are divided by the second, so that an arbitrary scale of blood flow per unit alveolar volume is obtained.

If only the distribution of ventilation is required, the lung can be scanned after a single breath of xenon. Again by rebreath-ing the xenon, complete equilibrium can be obtained in all alveoli. A scan taken at the end of a period of rebreathing, therefore, can be used as a measure of alveolar volume through-out the lung, and by comparing the two scans, ventilation per unit volume can be obtained.

The use of a number of individual counters or scanning techniques will no doubt ultimately give way to the gamma camera. In this instrument a large number of scintillation de-tectors are focused onto the organ or area of the body, and by the use of collimation each detector is arranged to 'see' only a small portion of the tissue. The number of counts recorded in each detector is scanned the whole time and may be reproduced as a pictorial record, with either intensity of dots, or changes in colour representing the mean counting rate from each individual detector. This will have enormous advantages over existing techniques. It is to be expected that such radioactive methods of studying pulmonary ventilation and blood flow will gradually become of increasing importance in clinical practice.

REFERENCES

BERNSTEIN L., D'SILVA J.L. & MENDEL D. (1952) The effect of the rate of breathing on the maximum breathing capacity determined with a new spirometer. *Thorax*, **7**, 255.

DYSON N.A., HUGH-JONES P., NEWBERRY G.R., SINCLAIR J.D. & WEST J.B. (1960) Studies of regional lung function using radioactive oxygen. *British Medical Journal*, **1**, 231.

EDMONDS–SEAL J. & MAROON J.C. (1969) Air embolism diagnosed with ultrasound. *Anaesthesia*, **24**, 438.

EGER E.I. & EPSTEIN R.M. (1964) Hazards of anesthetic equipment. *Anesthesiology*, **25**, 490.

HAGELSTEN J.O. & LARSEN O.S. (1965) Inaccuracy of anaesthetic flow-meters caused by static electricity. *British Journal of Anaesthesia*, **37**, 637.

HOBBS A.F.T. (1967) A comparison of methods of calibrating the pneumotachograph. *British Journal of Anaesthesia*, **39**, 899.

INGVAR D.H. & LASSEN N.A. (1961) Quantitative determination of regional cerebral blood flow in man. *Lancet*, **2**, 806.

KNIPPING H.W., BOLT W., VENRATH H., VALENTIN H., LUDES H. & ENDLER P. (1955) Eine neue Methode zur Prüfung der Herz- und Lungenfunction. *Deutsche Medizinische Wochenschrift*, **80**, 1146.

MCDOWALL D.G. (1964) Anaesthesia in a pressure chamber. *Anaesthesia* **19**, 321.

POWERS J.E. & SEVELIUS G. (1965) In: *Radioisotopes and Circulation*. 1st ed. (ed. Sevelius G.). Churchill, London.

SEVELIUS G. (1965) (ed.) *Radioisotopes and Circulation*. 1st ed. Churchill, London.

VEALL N. & MALLETT B.L. (1966) Regional cerebral blood flow determination by ^{133}Xe inhalation and external recording: the effect of arterial recirculation. *Clinical Science*, **30**, 353.

VISSCHER M.B. & JOHNSON J.A. (1953) The Fick principle: analysis of potential errors in its conventional application. *Journal of Applied Physiology*, **5**, 635.

WHITNEY R.J. (1953) The measurement of volume changes in human limb. *Journal of Physiology (London)*, **121**, 1.

WRIGHT B.M. & MCKERROW C.B. (1959) Maximum forced expiratory flow rate as a measure of ventilatory capacity. *British Medical Journal*, **2**, 1041.

FURTHER READING

HAMILTON W.F. & DOW P. (eds.) (1963) Blood flow through organs and tissues. In: *Handbook of Physiology*. Section II, Vol. II. Williams and Wilkins, Baltimore.

HARPER A.M. (1969) Measurement of cerebral blood flow. In: *Cerebral Circulation* (ed. D.G. McDowall). Little Brown, Boston.

INGVAR D.H. & LASSEN N.A. (1965) Methods for cerebral blood flow measurements in man. *British Journal of Anaesthesia*, **37**, 216.

McDOWALL D.G. (1969) Regional blood flow measurement in clinical practice. *British Journal of Anaesthesia*, **41**, 761.

PRYS-ROBERTS C. (1969) The measurement of cardiac output. *British Journal of Anaesthesia*, **41**, 751.

PUTMAN J.L. (1965) *Isotopes*. Penguin Books Ltd., Harmondsworth, Middlesex.

VEALL N. & VETTER H. (1958) *Radio-isotope Techniques in Clinical Research and Diagnosis*. Butterworth, London.

VEALL N. (1969) *Diagnostic Uses of Radioisotopes*. Hospital Medicine Publications, London.

WEST J.B. (1966) *U.K.A.E.A. Medical Monograph*. Radiochemical Centre, Amersham.

10

Measurement of Volume, Body Composition and Blood Loss

Measurement of volume is standardised in the S.I. system on the cubic metre. Water or mercury displacement and weighing is therefore the standard method of calibrating vessels which measure volume.

Measurements of gas volume are usually accomplished by collecting the gases in a calibrated spirometer, or by collecting the gases in a Douglas bag and then measuring the volume with a gas meter.

Spirometers

The standard spirometers (e.g. the 300 litre Tissot or the 6 litre Benedict–Roth) consist of a light cylinder which is suspended inside a larger double-walled container (Fig. 10.1). The space between the two walls is filled with water to form an air-tight junction. This type of spirometer is suitable for measurements at normal respiratory rates, but at high respiratory rates the inertia of the bell and pulleys and the fluctuations in water-level due to changes in pressure within the bell lead to inaccuracies. For recording at rapid respiratory rates a fast spirometer has been designed. This has a light bell of large diameter, which minimises the acceleration during rapid breathing, lightweight pulleys and chain and a large volume of water, which minimises oscillations (Bernstein, D'Silva & Mendel 1952).

Dry spirometers are more convenient for clinical work but are technically more difficult to construct. This type of spirometer utilises a freely moving bellows (which must be carefully folded so that the excursion is linearly related to volume) and this must be accurately counterbalanced by weights or springs so that the internal pressure is always close to atmospheric, whatever the contained volume.

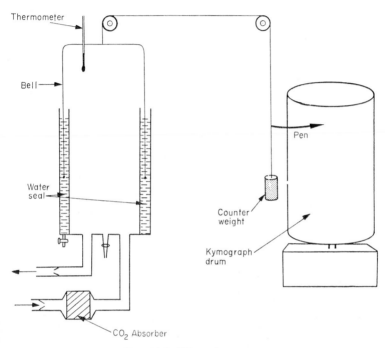

FIG. 10.1. Wet spirometer.

The Vitalograph is an example of this kind of instrument. The bellows is wedge shaped and its response is remarkably linear (Drew & Hughes 1969). Another type of dry spirometer has been described by Collins, McDermott & McDermott (1964).

Gas meters
Gas meters may be wet or dry. Wet meters are now rarely used since they need to be kept filled with water and carefully levelled: furthermore, the maximum flow rate which can be tolerated during measurement is limited to about 2·5 litres/min. Such a

meter consists essentially of a paddle-wheel, the lower half of which rotates under water. Gas is admitted to the space between two paddle blades and this causes the paddle to rotate. The gas then passes out through the exit tube. Since the volume of gas

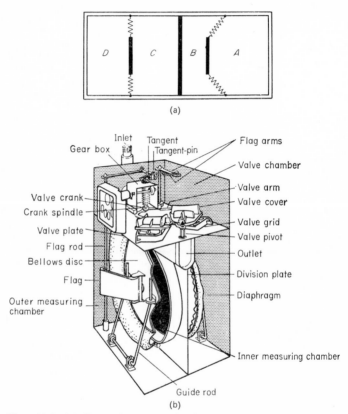

Fɪɢ. 10.2. (a) Coronal section of a dry gas meter. (b) Details of mechanism. (From Adams *et al.* 1967; reproduced by kind permission of the Editor of the *British Journal of Anaesthesia.*)

isolated in each section of the paddle-wheel is constant, the degree of rotation of the paddle-wheel is proportional to the volume flow. The paddle-wheel is connected to a gear chain which drives a pointer on a dial so that a direct reading is obtained.

Dry gas meters have found a much wider application in anaesthesia, since they are portable, accurate and relatively cheap. The meter consists of a box divided into two by a metal partition (Fig. 10.2). Each section of the box is further divided into two by a leather bellows. A rotary or sliding valve on the top of the meter is driven by arms attached to the bellows, and first directs the gas into chamber A. This bellows expands and later empties through the expiratory port. Gas then enters chamber B and the movement of the bellows is reversed. Chambers C and D are filled and emptied in a similar fashion but are 90° out of phase with chambers A and B. Since both leather partitions are attached to the valve mechanism, the drive originating from partition C/D will be maximal when the partition A/B is reversing its movement. This ensures smooth running and accurate measurements even at low flow rates. In addition to driving the valve mechanism, the movement of the bellows drives a pointer round a scale. The calibration of this scale can be accurately adjusted to match the excursion of the bellows by altering the length of a tangent arm on the valve mechanism. If properly adjusted and maintained these meters can be accurate to ±1 per cent over a range of flow rates from 0 to 100 litres/min (Adams *et al.* 1967).

The Dräger volumeter
This instrument is somewhat larger than the Wright respirometer (see below) and responds to airflow in either direction (Fig. 10.3). The registration of volume flow is accomplished by

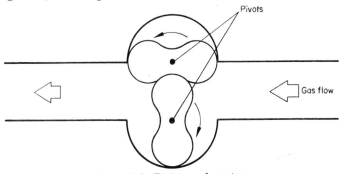

Fig. 10.3. Dräger volumeter.

two light, interlocking, dumb-bell-shaped rotors. The meter is more accurate than the Wright respirometer but also more expensive. It is affected by moisture but regains its accuracy when dried out.

Inferential meters

These are, in reality, flowmeters which have been calibrated to read in terms of volume, that is to say the volume is *inferred* from the flow rate.

Wright respirometer. This consists of a light mica vane which rotates within a small cylinder (Fig. 10.4). The wall of the cylinder is perforated with a number of tangential slits so that the air stream causes the vane to rotate. Flow in the reverse direction impinges on the bottom edge of the vane and so produces no rotational movement. The instrument is therefore unidirectional.

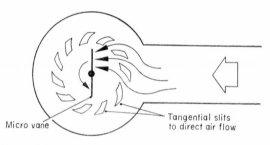

Micro vane

Tangential slits
to direct air flow

Fig. 10.4. Wright respirometer. Cross section (viewed from above).

The rotation of the vane activates a gear chain, which in turn drives the pointer round the dial. By adjusting the relation between the number of rotations of the vane and the volume of gas which has passed through the meter, it has been possible to arrange that the recorded volume approximates closely to the volume of gas which has actually passed through the meter. This calibration holds for normal tidal volumes and breathing rates, but the meter over-reads at high tidal volumes and under-reads at low tidal volumes. Similarly, the response to steady flow differs from that recorded during sinusoidal flow, and sinusoidal flow calibration differs from the calibration obtained with other waveforms (Byles 1960; Nunn & Ezi-Ashi 1962).

The instrument is delicate and is affected by the deposition of water vapour within it. It is also affected by the composition of the measured gas.

Ventigrator. This instrument was described by Maloney, Silverman & Whittenberger (1951) and investigated by Nunn & Ezi-Ashi (1962). The principle is that of the venturi flowmeter (Chapter 9), the pressure difference being proportional to the square of the gas flow. This results in marked insensitivity at low flow rates and high sensitivity at high flow rates. The volume scale is arbitrarily related to the pressure difference, so that volume is again inferred from flow rate. The pressure gauge is heavily damped so that a mean reading is obtained. The instrument is very sensitive to changes in the pattern of ventilation and to changes in gas composition, and has never found wide acceptance in clinical practice.

Pneumotachograph

This instrument (see page 125) may be used for volume measurement by integrating the flow signal with respect to time. This can be accomplished electronically with an integrator circuit (see Chapter 3).

Lung-function tests

Tests of lung function utilising measurements of pressure, flow and volume are detailed in Sykes (1967); Cotes (1968); Sykes, McNicol & Campbell (1969); and Nunn (1969).

BODY COMPOSITION

A body space is not an anatomical entity, but an abstraction which aids conceptual thinking. The composition of the body, the quantity of each component, and the size of the conceptual spaces are the result of many interrelated processes. Not only are they affected by the actual quantity of each component, but they depend on the rate of interchange between the various compartments and the rate of any losses or uptake.

For example, ^{131}I-labelled albumin may be used to measure the blood volume if a dilution sample is taken within a few minutes of the injection of the tracer. During this time the rate of loss of tracer is, normally, not significant. But over a longer period, the intravascular albumin comes into equilibrium with the total albumin pool, and the dilution of tagged albumin is no longer a valid measure of intravascular volume. Over a long period of time, the dilution of tracer gives a figure for the size of the albumin pool. If albumin is being lost in significant quantities while this slower equilibrium is being achieved, this invalidates the measurement of the total albumin pool.

Body composition can be measured in three fundamentally different ways: whole-body counting, neutron activation and dilution analysis.

Whole-body counting

Most elements occurring naturally consist of a mixture of isotopes (see Chapter 7), the majority of which are not radioactive. However, a small percentage may be radioactive, and if this is a fixed percentage of the total, an accurate count of the whole-body content of this isotope will indicate the total quantity of that ion present. The chief drawback is that to obtain an acceptable total number of counts, and therefore an acceptable level of accuracy, counting times may have to be unacceptably long.

Neutron activation analysis

The proportion of radioactive isotopes may be increased by bombarding the body with neutrons. When a bombarding neutron is captured, the capturing element becomes radioactive. The total number of captures is proportional to the amount of the substance present. This technique is at present being applied experimentally for the analysis of the body composition of a variety of ions.

Dilution analysis

If one starts with the assumption that there are no losses from the space being measured during the period of equilibration, then by applying the concept of the conservation of matter, the total quantity of diluted isotope is the same as the quantity injected. In the material being injected, this is the concentration (C) times the volume injected (v). In the dilution space, it is the volume of the space (V) plus the volume injected (v) times the concentration in the space (c). These total quantities are equal, i.e.:

$$C \times v = c(V + v)$$

The volume injected is small when compared with the dilution volume and may therefore be neglected. The equation then simplifies to:

$$V = \frac{C \times v}{c}$$

The concentrations of the injected tracer and dilution samples can be assayed by comparing their respective count rates under identical geometry. The semi-automated machines for measuring blood volume use a somewhat different approach (see below).

Although the equilibrium time for measuring blood volume is only a matter of minutes, the measurement of the extracellular space and of total body water require a much longer period of equilibration, about 3 hours for the extracellular space and up to 1 or 2 days for total body water. Changes in the dynamics of equilibration, and variations in intake and losses can make a big difference to the apparent results. When the dynamic situation is unstable, such as during and following major surgery, various alternative interpretations of the results achieved are always possible!

BLOOD VOLUME

Although a number of macabre methods have been used to estimate blood volume in the experimental animal, most human estimations have been performed with dye dilution or radio-isotope dilution methods.

Dye dilution
Blood volume may be measured using Evans blue as the tracer. A known dose is injected and a venous sample is withdrawn from the opposite arm after allowing a period of about 10 minutes

6*

for mixing to be complete. The concentration of dye in this sample is then estimated spectrophotometrically and from the relative concentrations of dye and the haematocrit the blood volume can be calculated (Albert 1963).

Semi-automated radioisotope dilution methods
Two instruments are in clinical use. The Volemetron is designed to measure blood volume with either ^{51}Cr-labelled red cells or ^{125}I or ^{131}I-iodinated human serum albumin. The Pitman Blood Volume Computer has been designed to measure blood volume using ^{125}I-iodinated human serum albumin.

All these isotopes are gamma-emittors, and the radiation is detected by scintillation detectors; ^{125}I, however, emits radiation of much lower energy. The shielding is consequently much less extensive and the instrument lighter and cheaper. Despite these differences, the operating principles of both instruments are similar.

A dose of isotope is suspended between two scintillation detectors and the total number of disintegrations detected over a fixed interval is recorded in a binary digital memory. This count, of course, includes some atmospheric background. After injection of the isotope into the patient, the container is counted again with the same geometry and for the same time, but any disintegrations detected are subtracted from the total in the memory. This also subtracts an equivalent amount of atmospheric background. After an appropriate interval, samples of blood containing diluted isotope are drawn from the patient. As the original dose is contained in about 1 ml, this represents a dilution of one in about four or five thousand. It would clearly be impractical to count these samples with the same geometry, although the time taken to detect the same number of counts from a similar volume of dilution sample would relate the dilution volume to the volume of tracer injected. To overcome this difficulty, the principle of geometrical equivalences has been deliberately abandoned. Dilution samples, although of fixed size, are bigger, and are counted in closer approximation to one of the counters, thereby greatly increasing the counting rate. The time taken to record the same number of counts is still the critical measurement, however, and this is utilised by making the detector subtract the counts from the memory until it reaches zero. The passage of time is observed by the movement of a pointer travelling at constant velocity across the scale. Now, the smaller the dilution volume, the more radioactive the samples will be. The more radioactive the samples, the shorter will be the time taken to empty the memory, and the less will be the distance the pointer will have travelled. It is thus possible to calibrate the dial directly in terms of volume. Calibration is achieved by adjusting the velocity of the dial needle so that a known dilution volume reads correctly. As this depends solely on the counting geometry, it can be done once and for all by the manufacturers. One essential refinement is that a sample of blood must be taken from the patient *before* the isotope is injected, in case there is any radioactivity present. This activity would contribute to a more rapid reduction in the memory counts, and to compensate for this, a similar sized pre-injection sample is counted simultaneously by the other detector with identical geometry and any disintegrations detected are *added* to the memory.

It should not be forgotten, that although these machines are called blood volume computers, they actually measure a dilution volume, usually an iodine-dilution volume. These are not necessarily comparable, since the sample of blood drawn from a peripheral vessel has a different haematocrit from the haematocrit of the whole body, and therefore does not contain a truly representative quantity of isotope. If the haematocrit of the sample is measured, and a normal value for the whole-body/venous haematocrit ratio is assumed, the true blood volume can be calculated. Failure to make this correction is only one of many errors in methodology that render the measurement of blood volume potentially very inaccurate (Heath & Vickers 1968).

Interpretation may be further complicated by sequestration of part of the circulating blood volume in states of shock or after cardio-pulmonary bypass. Nevertheless, the measurement of blood volume may prove useful when assessing a patient for surgery since blood volume is often reduced in cachectic conditions, after prolonged diuretic therapy and in patients with a phaeochromocytoma.

THE MEASUREMENT OF BLOOD LOSS

The volume-for-volume replacement of measured blood loss may prove inadequate when the preoperative blood volume is reduced, when there is an excessive loss of protein and fluid from the intravascular compartment, or when haemorrhage is concealed. Nevertheless the measurement of overt blood loss provides a useful guide to blood replacement: this can then be supplemented by an assessment of the clinical condition of the patient and with measurements of central venous pressure, urine output and mixed venous Po_2.

Suction loss

Suction loss is often difficult to measure accurately because of frothing or dilution with saline. If suction loss is large and the

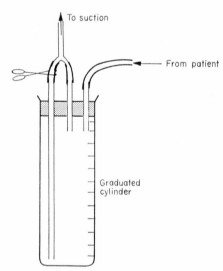

FIG. 10.5. Suction trap for accurate measurement of blood loss. If the clip is transferred to the opposite limb of the Y-piece the suction trap will be emptied to the main suction bottle.

degree of dilution is unknown an estimate of blood loss can be obtained by haemolysing the blood in the sucker and measuring the haemoglobin concentration or the electrical conductivity. The principles of these methods are discussed later.

In cardiac operations and in paediatric procedures it is often convenient to arrange for the volume of suction loss to be immediately indicated to the anaesthetist. This can be accomplished by using the apparatus shown in Fig. 10.5. It may be mounted at the head end of the table and may be emptied to the main suction reservoir at convenient intervals.

Direct inspection

With practice it is possible to make a rough estimate of blood loss by counting the number of swabs used. As a guide it may be assumed that the volume of blood on a swab is 5 ml if it is lightly stained, 10 ml if it is moderately stained and 15 ml if it is heavily stained (i.e. almost completely covered with blood). Abdominal packs hold a surprisingly large quantity of blood; indeed, three completely soaked abdominal packs will be equivalent to a loss of about 500 ml of blood.

Swab weighing

A millilitre of blood weighs approximately 1 g. If swabs are weighed before and after use it is possible to add swab loss to the volume of sucker contents to estimate total loss. Swab weighing has been greatly simplified by the use of pre-packed swabs of standard size. The used swabs are weighed in groups of five or ten and the weight of an equal number of dry swabs is subtracted either by simple arithmetic or by offsetting the scale on the balance. If a double-pan balance is used a pack of swabs may be placed on the weight pan to offset the swab weight on the other pan. Since drying will quickly reduce the weight of the blood on swabs it is important to weigh small groups of swabs at short intervals.

An alternative method which overcomes the drying error utilises trays containing water on each side of the balance. All contaminated swabs are placed in one tray as soon as they are used, and an equal number of clean swabs are then placed in the opposite tray. Since evaporation from the two trays occurs at equal rates the difference in weight between the two trays always indicates the blood loss.

Weighing is a less satisfactory method if the surgeon uses wet swabs. With practice nurses learn to squeeze swabs to a fairly constant degree of dryness, but even so large errors may occur.

Haemoglobin extraction–dilution

Various modifications of this technique have been suggested, but the basic principle is that the blood on the swabs is mixed with a large volume of diluent, either in a bucket or in a washing machine (Roe, Gardiner & Dudley 1962). If the volume of diluent is at least 100 times the volume of added blood and the haemoglobin of the shed blood and the blood-stained fluid are estimated, the volume of blood lost can be calculated, e.g.:

Volume of diluent = 100 litres
Hb of blood lost = 15 g per cent or 15×10 g/litre
Hb of blood and diluent = 0·2 g per cent = 2 g/litre
Then total quantity of Hb in 100 litres diluent = 2×100
  = 200 g

Therefore, blood loss $= \dfrac{200}{150} = 1\cdot33$ litre

This method is subject to a number of errors, the chief of which are the changing haematocrit during anaesthesia and surgery, faulty mixing and the size of the dead space in washing machines (Bond 1969). It is most suitable for losses below 1 litre, since bigger losses increase the dilution volume by a significant but unknown amount. For these reasons the method has not achieved great popularity.

Electrical conductivity

Blood lost is extracted into a volume of water as above, but the quantity of blood lost is calculated from the change in electrical conductivity of the diluent (LeVeen & Rubricius 1958). The electrical conductivity is measured by a Wheatstone bridge circuit, the conductivity cell forming one arm of the bridge. The instrument is bulky and expensive, and has not been widely used.

REFERENCES

ADAMS A.P., VICKERS M.D.A., MUNROE J.P. & PARKER C.W. (1967) Dry displacement gas meters. *British Journal of Anaesthesia*, **39**, 174.

ALBERT S.N. (1963) *Blood Volume*. C.C. Thomas, Springfield, Illinois.

BERNSTEIN L., D'SILVA J.L. & MENDEL D. (1952) The effect of the rate of breathing on the maximum breathing capacity determined with a new spirometer. *Thorax*, **7**, 255.

BOND A.G. (1969) Determination of operative blood loss. The sources of error and elimination of inaccuracy in the haemoglobin-dilution technique. *Anaesthesia*, **24**, 219.

BYLES P. (1960) Observations on some continuously acting spirometers. *British Journal of Anaesthesia*, **32**, 470.

COLLINS M.M., McDERMOTT M. & McDERMOTT T.J. (1964) Bellows spirometer and transistor timer for the measurement of forced expiratory volume and vital capacity. *Journal of Physiology (London)*, **172**, 39P.

COTES J.E. (1968) *Lung Function: Assessment and Application in Medicine*. 2nd ed. Blackwell Scientific Publications, Oxford and Edinburgh.

DREW C.D.M. & HUGHES D.T.D. (1969) Characteristics of the Vitalograph spirometer. *Thorax*, **24**, 703.

HEATH M.L. & VICKERS M.D. (1968) An examination of single tracer, semi-automated blood volume methodology. *Anaesthesia*, **23**, 659.

LeVEEN H.H. & RUBRICIUS J.L. (1958) Continuous, automatic, electronic determinations of operative blood loss. *Surgery, Gynecology and Obstetrics*, **106**, 368.

MALONEY J.V., SILVERMAN L. & WHITTENBERGER J.L. (1951) An integrating ventilation meter for clinical use. *Journal of Laboratory and Clinical Medicine*, **37**, 828.

NUNN J.F. & EZI-ASHI T.I. (1962) The accuracy of the respirometer and ventigrator. *British Journal of Anaesthesia*, **34**, 422.

NUNN J.F. (1969) *Applied Respiratory Physiology with Special Reference to Anaesthesia*. Butterworth, London.

ROE C.F., GARDINER A.J.S. & DUDLEY H.A.F. (1962) A simple instrument for continuous determination of operative blood loss. *Lancet*, **1**, 672.

SYKES M.K. (1967) Pulmonary compliance and airway resistance during anaesthesia. In: *Modern Trends in Anaesthesia*, Vol. 3, p. 56 (ed. F.T. Evans & T.C. Gray). Butterworth, London.

SYKES M.K., McNICOL M.W. & CAMPBELL E.J.M. (1969) *Respiratory Failure*. Blackwell Scientific Publications, Oxford and Edinburgh.

FURTHER READING

DAVIES J.W.L. (1966) Methods of assessment of blood loss in the shocked and injured patient. *British Journal of Anaesthesia*, **38**, 250.

MOORE F.D., OLESEN K.H., McMURREY J.D., PARKER H.V., BALL M.R. & BOYDEN C.N. (1963) *The Body Cell Mass and its Supporting Environment.* Saunders, Philadelphia.

THORNTON J.A., SAYNOR R., SCHROEDER H.G., TAYLOR D.G. & VEREL D. (1963) Estimation of blood loss with particular reference to cardiac surgery. *British Journal of Anaesthesia*, **35**, 91.

11
Gas Analysis

There are two main situations in which there is a need to analyse gases or vapours. The first is when it is necessary to test an anaesthetic machine, vaporizer or pipe-line installation. The second is in the assessment of lung function. In the latter situation it may be necessary to analyse the respired gases (oxygen, carbon dioxide and nitrogen) or to analyse a foreign gas which is used in one of the other tests of lung function (helium, carbon monoxide, etc.). In this chapter the commonest chemical and physical methods of gas analysis will be discussed. In general, the chemical methods remove fractional volumes from the gas phase by the production of non-gaseous compounds, the fractional concentration being determined by the reduction in volume which occurs. The physical methods, on the other hand, maintain the gas phase throughout and separate the fractions by utilising the atomic or molecular properties present.

CHEMICAL METHODS

The only chemical analyses which are likely to be carried out by the average anaesthetist are those for carbon dioxide and oxygen. It must be emphasised, however, that most physical methods of gas analysis need to be standardised with gas mixtures, the composition of which has been previously determined by chemical analysis.

Carbon dioxide

The concentration of CO_2 in gas mixtures is usually determined by measuring the reduction in volume after absorption of the gas in 10–20 per cent potassium hydroxide solution. This method cannot be used if another gas soluble in potassium hydroxide

167

(e.g. N_2O) is present. The difficulty can be overcome by allowing for the absorption of nitrous oxide during analysis (Glossop 1963) or by using saturated sodium hydroxide as the CO_2 absorbent (Nunn 1958). N_2O is relatively insoluble in the latter absorbent but the technique is difficult since the absorbent solution is extremely viscous and the precipitate of sodium carbonate which is formed obscures the meniscus.

Many pieces of apparatus have been described for carrying out this analysis; one of the most useful is the Campbell (1960)

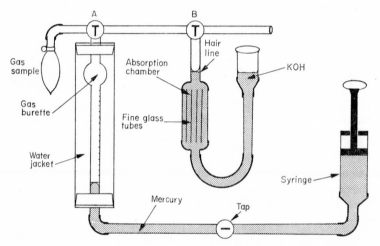

FIG. 11.1. Simplified CO_2 analyser (Campbell 1960).

modification of the Haldane apparatus (Fig. 11.1). This consists of a burette, absorption chamber and reservoir for the absorbent solution. The burette has a volume of 10 ml and the stem is graduated from 8·5 to 10 ml in 0·1 ml increments. Before starting the analysis the absorption chamber is opened to atmosphere and the absorbent reservoir is adjusted in height until the absorbent meniscus is exactly aligned with the hair line. This ensures that both columns of absorbent are exactly balanced when at atmospheric pressure.

The gas sample to be analysed is attached to the side limb of Tap A. A preliminary sample is aspirated into the burette, by raising the syringe plunger, and discharged to atmosphere through Tap B. Another sample is then aspirated into the burette and the excess gas is discharged through Tap B, exactly 10 ml being retained in the burette for analysis. (The 10 ml volume in this apparatus includes the volume in the cross-piece joining taps A and B.) The burette and absorption chamber are then connected by the appropriate adjustment of Taps A and B and the gas is driven to and fro between the gas burette and the absorption burette. After about ten to fifteen swings the absorbent meniscus is once again adjusted to the level of the hair line by manipulating the syringe plunger, and the reduction in the volume of gas in the burette is read off the mercury meniscus in the stem of the burette. The absorption process is repeated and the gas volume again checked to ensure that absorption is complete. Thus

$$\text{concentration of CO}_2 = \frac{\text{reduction in gas volume}}{\text{original volume}}$$

If the initial volume was exactly 10 ml, the concentration may be read directly from the figures engraved on the alternative scale on the right-hand side of the burette.

Care should be taken that the taps are well-lubricated and that the apparatus is free from leaks. The burette must be kept acidified with a few drops of dilute H_2SO_4 and the tube between the taps must be cleaned with a pipe-cleaner soaked in dilute H_2SO_4 if the KOH is accidentally drawn into it. The KOH should be replaced whenever absorption takes longer than twelve to fifteen swings. After a short period of practice most operators should be able to achieve duplicates within $\pm 0 \cdot 1$ per cent CO_2 (approximately 1 mmHg). A number of simpler, but less accurate, analysers are available (e.g. the Dräger and that described by Essex & Pask 1964).

Oxygen

The concentration of oxygen in a gas mixture can be determined in a similar fashion by absorbing the gas in alkaline pyrogallol or sodium anthraquinone. Since these solutions also absorb CO_2, the CO_2 analysis must be completed first. A standard Haldane apparatus with two absorption chambers is necessary. This apparatus has an additional burette which automatically compensates for changes in temperature during the analysis. The accuracy is therefore somewhat greater than the simplified apparatus ($CO_2 \pm 0.05$ per cent; $O_2 \pm 0.1$ per cent). Again, a number of simpler but less accurate methods are available (e.g. Pask 1959).

PHYSICAL METHODS

The main advantage of the physical methods of gas analysis is their speed. Indeed, they can often be adapted for continuous operation.

When a machine is designed to follow rapid changes in gas concentration it is essential to know the speed of response of

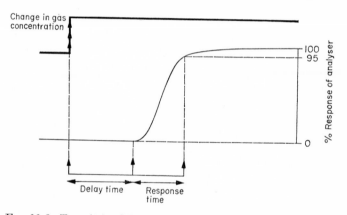

FIG. 11.2. Transit (or delay) time and rise (or response) time after a square wave change in gas concentration.

the complete system. This may be divided into two components (Fig. 11.2)—the time required for the sample to flow along the sampling catheter, and the time required for the instrument to react to the change in gas concentration. The former is often called the transit or delay time, whilst the latter is usually called the response or rise time. However, these terms are often used in different ways and some care is necessary when defining the causes of the total delay between a change in gas concentration and the inscription of the signal.

The transit time usually accounts for the greater part of the total delay. It is reduced by using a narrow and short sampling catheter with a rapid sampling rate. The response time of the instrument is chiefly due to the time required to wash out the analysis cell, but additional delays may be imposed by the mechanism used to detect the change in gas concentration. Commonly, the instrumental response to a square wave change in gas concentration is sigmoid in shape: it is therefore usual to express the instrumental response time as the time required to obtain a 90 or 95 per cent response to the change in gas concentration. If the response is exponential in character the time constant of the change can be quoted (Chapter 3). Ninety-five per cent response will then be achieved in three time constants.

Unfortunately, most physical methods of gas analysis utilise electronic circuitry and are therefore subject to zero drift and variations in sensitivity. For this reason physical methods often have to be calibrated frequently, either with a known input signal or with known gas mixtures; such mixtures can be manufactured accurately by special gas-mixing pumps. Alternatively, mixtures of the approximate concentration required may be decanting from other cylinders, and these may then be analysed by chemical methods. Vapour mixtures may be prepared by vaporising known weights of the liquid in known volumes of diluent gas.*

Physical methods of analysis may be classified into specific and non-specific methods according to the property of the gas which is used for analysis. Non-specific methods use a property of the gas which is common to all gases but possessed by each

* 1 gram-molecule of halothane vapour (molecular weight 197 g) occupies 22·4 litres at S.T.P.D. Therefore, 1 litre of halothane vapour weighs

$$\frac{197}{22\cdot4} = 8\cdot8 \text{ g}$$

To make a 2 per cent v/v concentration 8·8 g of halothane must be vaporized in 50 litres of air.

gas to a differing degree. Analysis of one gas can therefore only be conducted if the background is known and relatively constant. Examples of the properties used in non-specific methods are viscosity, density, thermal conductivity, refractive index, velocity of sound, and magnetic susceptibility. Specific methods utilise some property of the gas which is specific to that gas and so enables it to be identified in a gas mixture. Such methods may therefore be used when there are a number of background gases whose identity and concentration are unknown. Examples are the absorption and emission of radiation of a particular wavelength, atomic nuclear properties or the conduction of electricity in response to an applied voltage (polarography).

Non-specific methods

Density
This is one of the oldest methods employed and is chiefly of value in measuring the concentration of anaesthetic vapours which have a high vapour density. The principle was employed by Waller (1908) in his chloroform balance.

The principle of the balance is shown in Fig. 11.3. A sealed

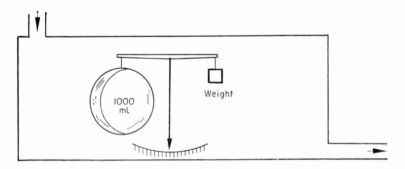

Fig. 11.3. Waller's chloroform balance.

glass bulb of about 1000 ml capacity is exactly counterbalanced by a small weight. If the glass bulb contains air and the background gas in the vapour mixture is air, then any decrease in weight of the glass bulb resulting from the admission of a vapour/air mixture to the cabinet must be due to the difference in weight between the vapour/air mixture and the air which it displaces. Now, 1000 ml of air weighs 1·3 g and 1000 ml of chloroform vapour weighs 5·3 g.* Hence the apparent reduction in weight when pure chloroform vapour is passed through the chamber is 5·3 − 1·3 = 4·0 g. If the reduction in weight is 0·04 g the vapour concentration must be 1 per cent. The scale on the balance can therefore be calibrated directly in terms of concentration. This technique is obviously most accurate when vapour density is high: it is essential that the background gas should remain constant.

Thermal conductivity

A gas with a high thermal conductivity conducts heat more readily than one with a low conductivity. This property is utilised in instruments known as katharometers. In these instruments the gas is passed over a heated wire. The degree of cooling of the wire depends on the temperature of the gas, the rate of gas flow and the thermal conductivity of the gas. The reduction in temperature of the wire alters its resistance, and so provides a signal which can be related to the gas concentration. The circuit is based on the Wheatstone bridge (Fig. 11.4), a current being passed through the resistors to heat them above ambient temperature. Resistors Q and S are placed in a cell which is flushed with the background gas of the mixture to be analysed. Resistors P and R are placed in a cell which is flushed with the gas to be analysed. The difference in thermal conductivity due to the presence of the analysis gas results in an alteration in the rate at which heat is conducted away from resistors P and R. These resistors therefore adopt a new temperature which represents the equilibrium between the heat being supplied by the electric current and the rate of heat loss.

---

* 1 gram-molecule of chloroform vapour occupies 22·4 litres at S.T.P.D. Therefore, 1 litre of vapour weighs

$$\frac{119}{22 \cdot 4} = 5 \cdot 3 \text{ g}$$

The change in resistance of P and R due to the change in temperature is measured by varying the value of the variable resistor on the Wheatstone bridge (Q') so as to bring the bridge back into balance. The value of this variable resistance can therefore be calibrated in terms of gas concentration. Alternatively, the output through the galvanometer may be used to drive a meter or recorder.

Katharometers can be made extremely sensitive and, by situating the resistors out of the main gas stream, they can be made relatively insensitive to changes of sample flow rate. The

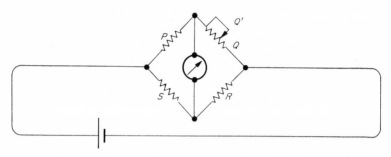

Fig. 11.4. Wheatstone bridge circuit used in thermal conductivity analyser. Resistance P and R are situated in the analysis cell and Q and S are in the reference cell. Q' is the variable resistor which may be adjusted to bring the bridge back into balance.

response time is then slow. If flow rate is rigidly controlled and the gas samples are passed through small (1 ml) analysis chambers a katharometer can be made to respond quickly to changes in gas concentration. Indeed, the response of some instruments is sufficiently rapid to permit breath-by-breath analysis of CO_2.

The use of this type of instrument is obviously dependent on the difference in thermal conductivity between analysis and background gas (Table 11.1). For example, the thermal conductivities of N_2 and O_2 differ by only 8 units in 589, and therefore analysis for one of these gases in the presence of the other is difficult. On the other hand, the apparatus can easily be used for the analysis of helium in nitrogen/oxygen mixtures, since a

TABLE 11.1. Properties of some common gases.

Gas	Molecular weight	Thermal conductivity (cal. cm^{-3} sec^{-2})	Sound velocity (m/sec)	Viscosity (micro-poise)
Air	28·8	583 × 10^{-7}	331	171
CO$_2$	44	352 × 10^{-7}	259	140
He	4	3480 × 10^{-7}	965	186
N$_2$	28	581 × 10^{-7}	334	165
N$_2$O	44	380 × 10^{-7}	263	135
O$_2$	32	589 × 10^{-7}	316	189

complete change of background gas from N_2 to O_2 would only produce a change equivalent to

$$\frac{8 \times 100}{3480} = 0\cdot23 \text{ per cent}$$

in measured helium concentration.

In clinical practice katharometers are usually used for the measurement of CO_2 and He, and are a useful and common form of detector for gas chromatography (see page 186).

Refractive index

Light passing through a gas experiences a phase retardation which is related to the refractive index of the gas and to the distance travelled through the gas. The degree of retardation also depends on the number of molecules present and so is affected by the pressure and temperature of the gas.

In the Rayleigh interference type of refractometer (Fig. 11.5a) light from a common source is collimated by a lens and passed through two vertical slits into two tubes, A and B. The tubes have plane-glass ends, and one tube (A) contains the gas or vapour to be analysed plus a background gas whilst the other (B) contains only background gas. The light beams pass out of the tubes and then fall onto two thin glass plates X and Y, each of which is inclined to the optical axis. The plate Y is fixed at an angle of about 45° to the optical axis, whilst the plate X can

be rotated about a horizontal axis which is mounted at an angle
of 90° to the optical path. Movement of this plate varies the

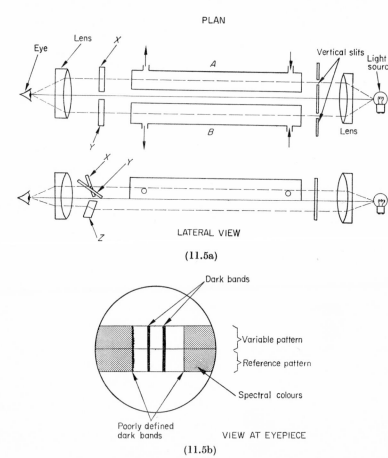

PLAN

LATERAL VIEW

(11.5a)

VIEW AT EYEPIECE

(11.5b)

Fig. 11.5. Refractive index method of gas analysis.

thickness of glass which is traversed by the beam passing
through tube A.

When the two tubes are filled with the same gas and X and
Y are inclined at the same angle to the optical path an interference pattern is produced. This appears at the eyepiece as a

spectrum (Fig. 11.5b) with a series of dark bands at its centre. If the gas in tube A is changed, the position of the interference bands is shifted. However, the shift can be counteracted by varying the thickness of glass in the light path by rotating X so that the interference bands once again appear in their original position. The degree of rotation of plate X can be measured with a vernier scale and calibrated to indicate the gas concentration in tube A.

In order to ensure that the interference pattern is correctly returned to the original position a duplicate pattern is reproduced below this movable pattern (Fig. 11.5b). This duplicate pattern is produced by the bottom half of the two beams of light produced by the collimator. These beams pass beneath the two tubes and are diverted by the prism Z, so that their interference pattern appears immediately below the other.

The instrument is mostly used for measurement of the concentration of one gas or vapour when the background gas is constant. It has been widely used in the calibration of vaporizers, since the calibration is stable and the reading can be quickly performed (Edmonson 1957).

Other types of direct-reading interferometers are used in industrial applications and are being investigated for possible use in anaesthesia.

Velocity of sound
There are a number of instruments which utilise this property in different ways. In one instrument (Stott 1957), the gas is resonated in a small chamber by an electronic circuit. The frequency of oscillation which causes the gas to resonate will depend on the velocity of sound in the gas mixture, and hence on the gas composition. This technique is most suitable when the cell volume must be kept small. In another instrument (Molyneux & Pask 1959) a pulse of sound is emitted at the end of two 1-metre tubes. One tube contains the gas mixture and the other the background gas. The difference in time taken by the sound to travel down the tubes gives a measure of the gas concentration. As can be seen from Table 11.1 the only gases of anaesthetic

interest with sound velocities widely different from air are carbon dioxide and nitrous oxide, although anaesthetic vapours can also be analysed by this technique.

Viscosity analyser

This type of analyser depends on the molecular weight and viscosity of a gas, and is commonly used for the analysis of CO_2 or He in air or oxygen. The flow of gas along a capillary tube

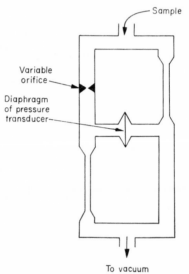

FIG. 11.6. Viscosity-type gas analyser.

is dependent on the viscosity of the gas, whereas flow through an orifice is practically independent of viscosity but dependent on molecular weight. These properties are utilised in the 'pneumatic Wheatstone bridge' arrangement shown in Fig. 11.6. By adjusting the size of the orifices it is arranged that the pressures on either side of the transducer diaphragm are equal when only the carrier gas flows. The addition of the gas to be analysed will then unbalance the bridge, so that a pressure difference is created across the transducer diaphragm. This can be calibrated by the use of suitable reference gases. This simple analyser has not been widely used in this country.

Magnetic susceptibility

Although this property is possessed by all gases, in practice only two gases, oxygen and nitric oxide, are strongly paramagnetic (i.e. attracted into a magnetic field). All other gases are weakly diamagnetic (i.e. repelled from such a field). The paramagnetism displayed by oxygen is so characteristic that the use of this property really falls into the category of specific methods of analysis. Nevertheless, it will be described in the present section.

The apparatus, in its simplest form, consists of a small chamber in the centre of a magnetic field. Inside the chamber are two small glass spheres which are connected by a bridge, the glass

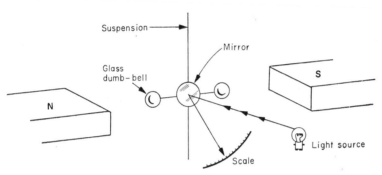

FIG. 11.7. Paramagnetic oxygen analyser.

dumb-bell which is so formed being suspended on a quartz thread. The glass spheres are filled with nitrogen and free to rotate around the axis of the quartz thread. The thread is tensed so that the resting position of the spheres is parallel to the main lines of force of the magnetic field (Fig. 11.7). If oxygen is now admitted to the chamber the oxygen molecules will be attracted to the centre of the magnetic field. They will therefore tend to force the glass spheres away from the centre of the field and the spheres will move in the only way possible, i.e. they will rotate around the axis formed by the quartz thread. The latter exerts a turning moment which attempts to return the glass spheres to their resting position: eventually a point of balance is reached at which the two turning moments are equal. The deflection of the glass spheres may be recorded by attaching a small mirror and noting the position of a reflected light beam on a scale. Alternatively the glass spheres may be brought back to their resting position by the application of an opposing magnetic field. The use of this null deflection technique enables the accuracy to be increased from ± 1 or 2 per cent to $\pm 0\cdot 1$ per cent O_2. Water vapour greatly affects paramagnetic O_2 analysers, so that all gases must be dried by passage through silica gel before entering the analysis chamber. If extreme accuracy is required a small correction for diamagnetic gases present in the background gas must be made.

The two outstanding British examples of this type of instrument have been evaluated by Nunn *et al.* (1964) and Ellis & Nunn (1968).

Specific methods

Emission of electromagnetic radiation

If suitably excited, all gases will emit electromagnetic radiation in some part of the ultra-violet, visible or infra-red portions of the spectrum, the fluorescent lighting tube being a common example of this phenomenon. This principle has been used in a number of gas analysers, the most familiar example being the nitrogen meter. This is used in tests of respiratory function such as the single-breath method of measuring anatomical dead space and the nitrogen washout test for assessing the distribution of ventilation.

A powerful suction pump draws the gas sample through a fine needle valve (placed close to the patient) to a gas discharge tube (Fig. 11.8). Two electrodes are sealed into the ends of this tube and a potential of about 1500–2000 volts is applied. This ionises the gas, which glows, the wavelength of the radiation emitted being characteristic of the gas. A reflector placed behind the tube directs the light through a filter (which eliminates all but the desired wavelengths) onto a photo-electric cell. This cell produces a current which is proportional to the intensity of the radiation falling on it, and this current is then amplified and displayed on a meter.

The great advantage of the N_2 meter is its specificity and rapid response. The transit time from needle valve to discharge tube and the time required to wash out the tube are minimised by the reduction in pressure in the system, and the delay time and response time are accordingly very short, the total delay being in the order of 20–40 milliseconds.

Unfortunately, the light output from the gas discharge tube and, therefore, the electrical output from the photo-electric cell, is alinear, and linearising circuits have to be added. This makes

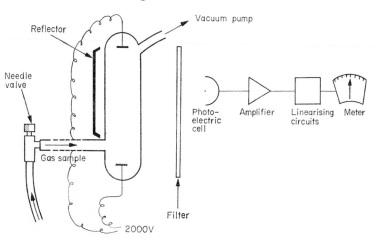

Fɪɢ. 11.8. Nitrogen meter.

the machine expensive. Attempts to analyse other common gases with this technique have not been exploited commercially, because of weak emission spectra.

Absorption of radiation

All gases are also capable of absorbing electromagnetic radiation, the wavelengths most commonly used for this purpose being in the infra-red and ultra-violet regions of the spectrum.

Infra-red gas analysers. Infra-red radiation is absorbed by all gases with more than two atoms in the molecule. If there are only two atoms, absorption will only occur if the two atoms are dissimilar. Thus O_2 does not absorb infra-red radiation.

The instruments used in this type of analysis may be classified as dispersive or non-dispersive.

The infra-red spectrometer is an example of the dispersive type of analyser. In this instrument radiation from an infra-red source passes through a prism or diffraction grating and is so dispersed that the radiations of different wavelengths are arranged in sequence. If now the gas to be analysed is placed in

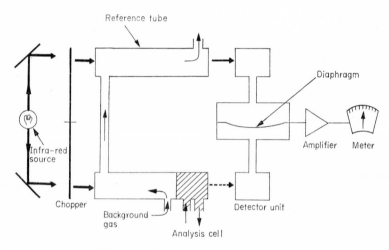

FIG. 11.9. Infra-red gas analyser.

the path of the radiation it will absorb maximally in one or more regions of the spectrum. By scanning the whole spectrum a graph of wavelength against absorption can be plotted. Alternatively, the absorption at a particular wavelength can be studied. This type of instrument is versatile and can readily be adjusted for measurements on different gases which have different absorption spectra. It is, however, expensive and if interest is centred on only one gas the non-dispersive type of analyser is often used. In this instrument (Fig. 11.9) light from an infra-red source (yielding a wide range of wavelengths) is directed down two tubes whose ends are sealed with quartz or a similar substance which transmits infra-red radiation. The gas sample to be analysed is circulated through the analysis cell, whilst the remainder of the tube on this side, and the reference tube, is flushed with air or other background gas. The gas in the analysis cell absorbs a small proportion of the infra-red radiation and the strength of the radiation impinging on the detector is therefore less than that impinging on the detector on the reference side.

The Luft type of detector is now commonly used. This consists of two chambers containing the gas or vapour to be analysed. The gas in the chambers also absorbs the infra-red radiation, and is therefore heated. This causes the gas to expand. The detector on the reference side receives more radiation than that on the analysis side and the difference in pressure in the two chambers is measured by recording the deflection of the elastic membrane separating them. This part of the detector is therefore a pressure transducer, the capacitance principle being the method most commonly used. To prevent drift due to slow heating of the detector cells the light from the infra-red source is 'chopped' by a rotating shutter so that it cycles on/off at a frequency of about 25 Hz. This produces an alternating output from the transducer which is then amplified and displayed.

Unfortunately, there are two sources of error in this technique. In the first place there is often some overlap in the absorption wavebands of different gases (Fig. 11.10). The background gas may therefore absorb some of the infra-red radiation, so causing an over-estimate of the concentration of the gas to be analysed. This error can be overcome by flushing the remainder of the analysis tube and the reference tube with the background gas. A second error arises from the phenomenon of 'collision broadening'. This causes the absorption spectrum to become broader, with the result that the degree of overlap varies with the gas concentrations. Corrections to measured gas concentrations have been published (Stow 1952; Cooper 1957; Ramwell & Dawson 1958; Severinghaus, Larson & Eger 1961), but the simplest method of eliminating this error is to calibrate the instrument with gas mixtures which contain the same background gas as that to be analysed.

7

By suitable adjustment of cell size and sample rate this type of analyser can be made sufficiently quick in response (150–300 milliseconds) to permit breath-by-breath analysis. In addition to its use in measuring CO_2 this type of analyser has been used for the analysis of ether, halothane, alcohol and many other vapours.

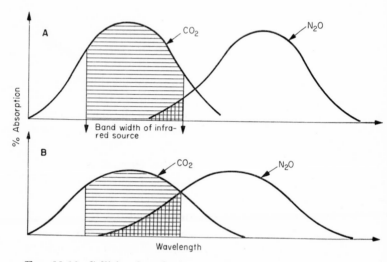

FIG. 11.10. Collision broadening. A. The absorption spectra of CO_2 and N_2O when plotted independently. B. The increased overlap of the absorption spectra due to collision broadening.

Ultra-violet analysis. Analysis in the ultra-violet region of the spectrum has been mainly used in connection with the analysis of halothane (Robinson, Denson & Summers 1962). Such a meter is relatively cheap and quite stable if allowed to warm up for at least an hour. The response time of commercial instruments is generally slow, but the instrument can be modified to provide a more rapid response.

Mass spectrometer

As its name implies, this machine splits each gas in a mixture into a spectrum which is based on the mass of the various particles present. A small proportion of the gas sample (about 15 ml/min) is drawn into an evacuated ionisation chamber through a molecular leak. In the chamber the gas molecules are bombarded by a stream of electrons, the charged particles then being accelerated out of the chamber in the form of a narrow stream. The charged particles are next separated by deflecting them into an arc by means of a magnetic field (Fig. 11.11). The lighter ions are deflected most and the heaviest least. Each stream of ions is then sampled by a detector, the signal being amplified and displayed

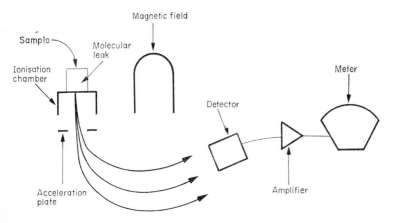

FIG. 11.11. The mass spectrometer.

to indicate the number of ions of that particular mass number in the mixture. Commonly, instead of providing a separate detector for each gas stream one detector is used to sample each stream in turn. This is accomplished by sweeping the spectrum to and fro across the detector about twenty-five times per second by varying the voltage on the accelerator plate. The output from the detector is then scanned intermittently, so that the output from each individual gas stream is fed to the appropriate channel in the display and recording apparatus.

It might be expected that such an instrument would be unable to separate two gases with the same mass numbers (e.g. CO_2 and N_2O, both of which have a mass number of 44). In practice a high proportion of the molecules are fragmented during the process of ionisation so that it is possible to monitor some other fraction such as NO (mass weight = 30). The mass spectrometer is extremely versatile and is widely used in the petroleum industry for separating complex mixtures. It has a rapid response and, although expensive and bulky, has proved invaluable in laboratories devoted to respiratory problems.

Gas chromatography
This is a contraction for gas–liquid chromatography, a term which is not in itself, at first sight, fully explanatory. Indeed the purist will never be able to reconcile the implications of colour in 'chromatography' with the separation of totally colourless gases and vapours. The terminology has been inherited from the older separation technique of liquid–liquid chromatography, in which the separated components were identified by their respective colours, either natural or induced by chemical treatment.

The essential element of all chromatographic techniques is the partition of substances between two solvents. One of these solvents is adsorbed onto an inert material and is referred to as the stationary phase. In gas–liquid chromatography, the stationary phase is a liquid organic solvent adsorbed onto an inert material such as firebrick dust. The stationary phase used depends on the nature of the substances which are to be separated, and is chosen by reference to the relative solubilities of these substances in the stationary phase *vis-à-vis* their solubility in the moving phase. In gas–liquid chromatography the moving phase is, of course, gaseous, and the components of the mixture must therefore be in the gaseous state. This may involve heating the column considerably throughout its length, or of heating an initial portion to drive gases out of solution or chemical combination. To maintain the flow down the column, the components are 'dissolved', as it were, in a large volume of continuously flowing 'solvent' gas, usually called the carrier gas.

The column is usually only a few millimeters in diameter, is made of stainless-steel tubing, and varies in length from a few inches to many feet. When the carrier gas flows along it carrying the substances for analysis, there is a time delay between the entry and exit of any substance, and this time delay, because it depends on the solubility of the compound in the stationary phase, is different for every component of the mixture. The actual transit time depends on numerous variables, such as the gas flow rate, the temperature of the column, the length of column and the actual stationary phase employed. Consequently, all such variables must be rigidly controlled if consistent results are to be obtained.

If the column is too short, or the solubility of the compound in the stationary phase is low, there is a rather indefinite spread of the emerging compound. If the compound has no affinity for the stationary phase it is not subject to delay and so will emerge with other compounds having similar characteristics.

So far it will be clear that the only function of the chromatograph column is to separate the components of a mixture. Before the technique can be of any practical use, it is necessary to be able to identify which compound is which, and then to measure their relative concentrations. These are the functions of the detector.

The detector is designed to signal the presence of any substance other than the carrier gas, and to produce a signal proportional to the mass of that substance. There are several types of detectors, and again the choice depends on the substances being detected. The simplest is a thermal conductivity detector or katharometer. This is a heated thermistor which, in a constant stream of carrier gas, assumes a steady temperature when the heat supplied is balanced by heat loss. When a gas or vapour with a different thermal conductivity arrives at the detector, this balance is upset. The change of temperature associated with the change of electrical resistance of the thermistor can be measured by making the detector one limb of a Wheatstone bridge circuit. This, therefore, yields an output which is dependent on the concentration of the compound present.

If such a detector is used, its sensitivity will depend on how much the thermal conductivity of the substance being measured differs from the thermal conductivity of the carrier gas. The thermal conductivity of helium differs widely from many of the gases commonly analysed, so that it is often used as the carrier gas.

The presence of organic compounds can be detected with great sensitivity by using a flame ionization detector. Here, the carrier gas is hydrogen which is ignited between electrically charged plates in the detector. Organic compounds yield ionized products when heated in this flame, and these migrate in the electrostatic field and alter the voltage on the plates. Halogenated compounds can be identified with even greater sensitivity by an electron capture detector. In this device the emerging components are bombarded by gamma-rays from a small quantity of long-life isotope and the electrons emitted from the halogen ions are collected electrically.

Although the detector is able to signal the arrival of something that is not carrier gas, it is still necessary to identify the substance.

If the likely components of the mixture are known, or if only a few are of any interest, each one can be injected individually into the column and its appearance time noted. Provided that the column conditions are not altered this time will remain constant, and so any component of a mixture which has the same appearance time must be that substance.

The final problem is the measurement of the concentration of the various substances. Since the sensitivity of the detector is different for each component, no absolute calibration is possible. It is necessary to inject an accurately known quantity of the substance, and observe the signal produced. The quantity should be of the same order as the mass of that substance expected in the sample during the course of a run.

This is not always feasible and there is an alternative method, in which a known amount of another substance is added to each sample before it is injected into the column. This relies on the fact that the relative sensitivities of the standard and test substance will be unchanged, even if column conditions, gas flow, or amplifier gain happen to alter. If the column has once been calibrated for this internal standard and the test substance, the concentration of the latter can be derived by comparing the reading of the standard with its calibration.

The electrical output of a detector is proportional to the mass of the substance passing through the detector at that instant. If the sample size is fixed, concentrations can be derived. The output appears as a deflection from the base line, and if this is drawn on a paper moving at constant speed, the area between the curve and the base line is proportional to the total mass of that compound in the sample. If the chromatographic separation is good, the deflection has an abrupt onset, short duration, and abrupt termination, and appears as a peak. Under these conditions, the peak bears a close approximation to a triangle, and the area can be found as

$$\frac{\text{half height}}{\text{base}}$$

or more commonly, height times width at half height (since the base may be distorted by contaminants). If the base is always the same, then the peak height alone is proportional to area, and is an acceptable simplification. However, where peaks are broad, area must be measured. It goes without saying, that ideally the peaks from each component of the mixture should not overlap; if they do, there are various methods of computing what their area would be without the presence of the overlapping peak.

Many chromatographs can be fitted with a mechanical system called a disc integrator. The basis of the device is a flat disc, rotating at constant speed, on the centre of which is suspended a ball. As long as the ball is in the dead centre, it will not rotate, but if it moves outwards on the disc it will revolve at a velocity which increases the further it moves towards the rim. The movement of the ball across the disc is geared to the movement of the pen which is tracing the chromatogram. The rotation of the ball is geared to another writing system, which traces out a series of deflections, each one representing a number of revolutions. The number of revolutions is proportional to area, since the speed increases the further the trace is from the base line, and both quantities are multiplied by time.

Finally, it is possible to integrate the area electrically (see Chapter 3).

Polarography

If two electrodes are connected by a buffered electrolyte and a potential of about 0·6 volts is maintained between them it is found that the current which flows is proportional to the concentration of oxygen present in the electrolyte. By imprisoning a thin layer of electrolyte under a membrane the electrode can be made to respond to changes in oxygen concentration on the other side of the membrane. This is the basis of the oxygen electrode (Chapter 12).

Radioactive isotopes

Gases can be 'labelled' by incorporating radioactive isotopes in the mixture. This enables their fate in the body to be followed with great accuracy. There are many technical difficulties associated with this type of work, but the principle has now been widely used in respiratory physiology and has contributed greatly to our knowledge of the distribution of pulmonary ventilation and blood flow (see Chapter 10).

REFERENCES

CAMPBELL E.J.M. (1960) Simplification of Haldane's apparatus for measuring CO_2 concentration in respired gases in clinical practice. *British Medical Journal*, **1**, 457.

COOPER E.A. (1957) Infrared analysis for the estimation of carbon dioxide in the presence of nitrous oxide. *British Journal of Anaesthesia*, **29**, 486.

EDMONSON W. (1957) Gas analysis by refractive index measurement. *British Journal of Anaesthesia*, **29**, 570.

ELLIS F.R. & NUNN J.F. (1968) The measurement of gaseous oxygen tension utilizing paramagnetism: an evaluation of the 'Servomex' 0.A150 analyser. *British Journal of Anaesthesia*, **40**, 569.

ESSEX L. & PASK E.A. (1964). A simple CO_2 gas analyzer. Lancet, **1**, 311.

GLOSSOP M.W. (1963) A simple method for the estimation of carbon dioxide concentration in the presence of nitrous oxide. *British Journal of Anaesthesia*, **35**, 17.

MOLYNEUX L. & PASK E.A. (1959) A sonic analyser for anaesthetic vapours. *Anaesthesia*, **14**, 191.

NUNN J.F. (1958) Respiratory measurements in the presence of nitrous oxide. *British Journal of Anaesthesia*, **30**, 254.

NUNN J.F., BERGMAN N.A., COLEMAN A.J. & CASSELLE D.C. (1964) Evaluation of the Servomex paramagnetic oxygen analyser. *British Journal of Anaesthesia*, **36**, 666.

PASK E.A. (1959) An oxygen analyser. *Lancet*, **2**, 273.

RAMWELL P.W. & DAWSON J.B. (1958) Calibration of infra-red gas analysers for use in the estimation of carbon dioxide. *Physics in Medicine and Biology*, **2**, 280.

ROBINSON A., DENSON J.S. & SUMMERS F.W. (1962) Halothane analyzer. *Anesthesiology*, **23**, 391.

SEVERINGHAUS J.W., LARSON C.P. & EGER E.I. (1961) Correction factors for infrared carbon dioxide pressure broadening by nitrogen, nitrous oxide and cyclopropane. *Anesthesiology*, **22**, 429.

STOTT F.D. (1957) Sonic gas analyzer for measurement of CO_2 in expired air. *Review of Scientific Instruments*, **28**, 914.

STOW R.W. (1952) Systematic error in infrared analysis for carbon dioxide in respiratory gas mixtures. *Federation Proceedings*, **11**, 155.

WALLER A.D. (1908) The chloroform balance. A new form of apparatus for the measured delivery of chloroform vapour. *Journal of Physiology (London)*, **37**, 6P.

FURTHER READING

HILL, D.W. & POWELL T. (1968) *Non-dispersive Infra Red Gas Analysis in Science, Medicine and Industry*. Adam Hilger Ltd., London.

WORTLEY D.J., HERBERT P., THORNTON J.A. & WHELPTON D. (1968) The use of gas chromatography in the measurement of anaesthetic agents in gas and blood. *British Journal of Anaesthesia*, **40**, 624.

12

pH and Blood-Gas Analysis

In conscious patients with normal lungs the alveolar gas has a P_{CO_2} close to that of the arterial blood. The analysis of an end-tidal sample by chemical or physical methods will thus provide a reasonable estimate of arterial P_{CO_2}. During anaesthesia there is an arterial-to-alveolar CO_2 tension difference of about 5 mmHg due to an increase in alveolar dead space: when the arterial P_{CO_2} is 40 mmHg the end-tidal CO_2 concentration will therefore be about 5 per cent. In patients with lung disease the arterial-to-alveolar P_{CO_2} difference may increase to 10–20 mmHg. This renders the method quite inaccurate. For this reason, the continuous analysis of expired gas or the analysis of discrete end-tidal samples is of most value when it is desired to monitor rapid changes of P_{CO_2} in patients with relatively normal lungs.

The use of the rebreathing technique, in which equilibrium is established between gas in a reservoir bag and the mixed venous P_{CO_2}, overcomes the problem imposed by the increased CO_2 tension difference resulting from an enlarged dead space and is particularly useful when repeated measurements are required at short time intervals. It is, however, subject to errors arising from leaks and incomplete equilibration. Furthermore, in patients with a low cardiac output, there is an increase in the normal venous-to-arterial P_{CO_2} difference. The assumption of a 6 mmHg venous-to-arterial difference may therefore lead to an overestimate of arterial P_{CO_2}.

The calculation of P_{CO_2} from pH and bicarbonate concentration using the Henderson–Hasselbalch equation is now rarely used, since it has been found that pK′ varies with pH and temperature. This error, plus the known errors of pH measurement, renders the method too inaccurate for general use. There are situations, however, in which the bicarbonate or total CO_2 content may have already been determined on an autoanalyser but in which the respiratory status may be unknown. A single pH measurement may then provide sufficient information to enable a diagnosis to be made. Repeated pH measurements over a period of 1–2 hours may also be used to assess the result of therapy in respiratory disorders, on the assumption that the non-respiratory component is unlikely to change greatly over such a short period of time. This may prove useful if the blood-gas laboratory is overloaded or the doctor is performing the analyses himself.

The indirect estimation of arterial $P\text{co}_2$ by the Astrup interpolation technique is much more accurate than the use of the Henderson–Hasselbalch equation, since the slope of the buffer line is determined on each blood sample. It also has the advantage that the non-respiratory component of acid-base balance is determined as well. It is, however, subject to the error resulting from the difference between the *in vitro* and *in vivo* buffer lines, and there are also a number of other possible errors in the technique which can summate.

The CO_2 electrode provides the most accurate method of determining blood $P\text{co}_2$, although this again is an indirect technique, since it involves determining the pH of a bicarbonate solution which has been equilibrated with the blood sample. The direct chemical analysis of a gas bubble which has been equilibrated with the blood sample (Riley technique) cannot be carried out in the presence of an anaesthetic gas, is technically very difficult and is now rarely used. It was, however, for many years the only method of directly determining CO_2 tension.

Rebreathing methods
There are many variations on the basic method, but the successful application of the technique depends more on a thorough understanding of the principles than on the actual technique employed.

The method is based on the discovery by Plesch (1909) that the rebreathing of a suitable gas mixture will lead to its equilibration with mixed venous blood. As pointed out by Hackney, Sears & Collier (1958), the venous-to-arterial $P\text{CO}_2$ difference is remarkably constant at about 6 mmHg and therefore, if the mixed venous $P\text{CO}_2$ is determined, the arterial $P\text{CO}_2$ can easily be calculated. The two main problems in the technique are first, to ensure that complete equilibrium between the gas in the bag, lungs and mixed venous blood is attained before recirculation occurs and second, to maintain adequate oxygenation of the

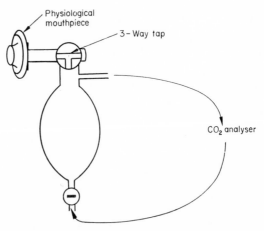

Fig. 12.1. Reservoir bag, 3-way tap and mouthpiece used for rebreathing technique. Intermittent samples are normally removed through the tail of the bag. If a continuous analyser is used an additional sample point is required.

patient during the procedure. The following technique, described originally by Campbell & Howell (1962) and modified by Godfrey (1965), has been found to be of most value.

A 2-litre reservoir bag fitted with a tap and face mask or physiological mouth-piece is half filled with oxygen (Fig. 12.1). The mask is applied tightly to the face (to prevent leaks) and at the end of a normal expiration the tap is opened so that the patient can rebreathe into the bag. The patient is encouraged to breathe deeply so that adequate mixing is obtained between the gas in the lungs and the bag. After about 30–60 seconds most patients begin to hyperventilate. When this occurs, or after 90 seconds rebreathing if it does not, the patient is disconnected from the bag, the tap being turned so that the last expiration is retained in the bag. Since recirculation of blood will have occurred during the rebreathing procedure, this gas mixture should have a P_{CO_2} which is 7–14 mmHg higher than the patient's original mixed venous P_{CO_2}. A check analysis of the composition of this gas can be made.

After a rest of 2–3 minutes, during which the patient eliminates the excess CO_2 retained during the rebreathing procedure, the patient is again connected to the bag. Rebreathing is continued for 20–25 seconds (i.e. six to ten breaths) and the bag is again disconnected at the end of an expiration and analysed. This sample should have the same P_{CO_2} as mixed venous blood. Since appreciable recirculation should not have occurred, the subtraction of 6 mmHg from this value should yield arterial P_{CO_2}.

To check that equilibration is complete it is as well to perform a third period of rebreathing of 30–40 seconds duration. Some recirculation will occur during this period, but since the rate of rise of P_{CO_2} in the apnoeic patient (i.e. one not eliminating CO_2) is about 3–5 mmHg/min, the bag P_{CO_2} at the end of the third period of rebreathing should be no more than 1–3 mmHg higher than the previous value. If the P_{CO_2} is more than 4 mmHg above the previous value it suggests that the initial period of rebreathing was too short and that the P_{CO_2} of the gas in the bag at the beginning of the second period of rebreathing was so low that complete equilibration with mixed venous blood could not be achieved in the time available. Reference to the analysis of the bag contents at the end of the first period of rebreathing will confirm this. If the P_{CO_2} falls after each of the three periods of rebreathing it suggests that the initial period of rebreathing was continued for too long and that the initial gas mixture had too high a P_{CO_2}. This pattern is rare. Gross departures from these two patterns suggest that leaks have vitiated the procedure, and it should therefore be repeated.

The procedure should ideally be monitored by a rapid CO_2 analyser (Fig. 12.2). The attainment of equilibrium during the first and second rebreathing periods can then be detected by direct observation of the trace, and the third period of rebreathing becomes unnecessary. If such an analyser is not available, perfectly satisfactory results can be obtained by analysis of gas samples from the bag with the Campbell modification of the Haldane apparatus (page 168). If nitrous oxide is present the CO_2 electrode must be used, since nitrous oxide is soluble in potassium hydroxide.

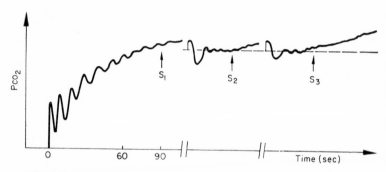

FIG. 12.2. CO_2 concentration as sampled at the mouth during the rebreathing method for determining mixed venous Pco_2. The three periods of rebreathing are separated by intervals during which the patient eliminates the CO_2 retained during the rebreathing procedure. The arrows S_1, S_2, S_3 indicate the times of sampling when chemical analysis is used.

The rebreathing technique can be used successfully with apnoeic patients and with children (Sykes 1960). It may, however, prove somewhat inaccurate in patients with a marked reduction in cardiac output, since the venous-to-arterial Pco_2 difference may then increase to 10 or 15 mmHg. With this exception an accuracy of ± 3 mmHg should be readily obtainable.

Astrup interpolation technique
This technique is based on the observation that there is an almost linear relationship between the pH and log Pco_2 of any particular blood sample over the physiological range, pH falling as Pco_2

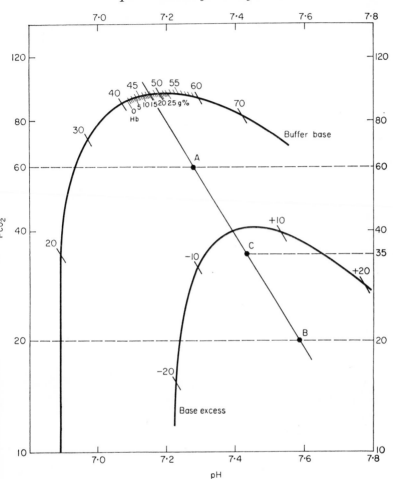

Fig. 12.3. Principle of Astrup interpolation technique plotted on Siggaard-Andersen nomogram (1962). Points A and B are obtained by measuring the pH of two samples of the patient's blood which have equilibrated with two O_2–CO_2 gas mixtures of known P_{CO_2} (in this case 60 and 20 mmHg). Point C is interpolated from the measured pH of the patient's blood. The P_{CO_2} can then be read off the ordinate. The base excess (zero) is read from the lower curve. In a non-respiratory alkalosis the buffer line A–B is shifted to the right and in a non-respiratory acidosis it is shifted to the left.

is increased (Fig. 12.3). The line obtained by plotting the pH readings against the relevant $P\text{co}_2$ values (plotted on a logarithmic scale) represents the buffer line of that particular blood sample. The slope of the line depends on the buffering power of the blood and hence on the concentration of plasma proteins and haemoglobin. The changes in plasma proteins encountered in clinical practice have little effect, so that the slope of the line depends predominantly on haemoglobin concentration, the slope being steepest when the haemoglobin concentration is high.

The position of the line in relation to the ordinate depends on the non-respiratory state of the blood sample, the line being displaced to the left if there is a non-respiratory (or metabolic) acidosis and to the right if there is a non-respiratory alkalosis. Three scales are provided on the nomogram to enable the non-respiratory component to be quantified. The *base excess* curve indicates the change in pH which would occur if increments of acid or base were added to a normal sample of blood. Thus the addition of 5 mEq/litre of acid would result in a *base deficit* of 5 mEq/litre, or a *base excess* of −5 mEq/litre whilst the addition of 5 mEq/litre of alkali would result in a base excess of +5 mEq/litre. This measure of the non-respiratory component is independent of haemoglobin concentration since the curve represents the points at which the buffer lines of blood of different haemoglobin concentration, but equal base deficit or excess, intersect (Fig. 12.4). This measure of the non-respiratory component greatly simplifies the task of correcting any abnormality which is present, since it gives a direct indication of the quantity of acid or base which must be added to correct the deficit. The second scale commonly shown is the *standard bicarbonate*. This represents the bicarbonate concentration of the plasma of the blood sample when it has been equilibrated with an O_2–CO_2 gas mixture of $P\text{co}_2 = 40$ mmHg at 37°C. Since this value refers to plasma bicarbonate, any deficit in base will only be made good if the dose of bicarbonate given is 1·1 to 1·2 times the deficit in standard bicarbonate. The third scale is that referring to *buffer base*. The normal buffer base depends on the haemoglobin concentration, since it represents the total quantity of buffer anions present in the sample. The normal buffer base value for each haemoglobin concentration is shown by reference to the haemoglobin scale situated on the buffer base curve. If the

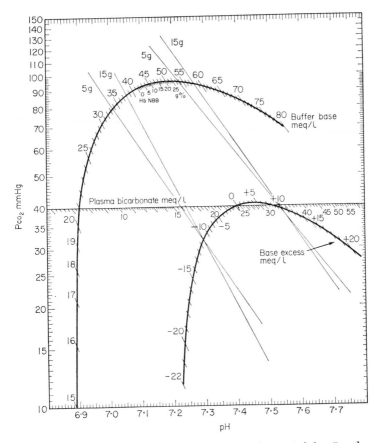

FIG. 12.4. Buffer lines for normal blood samples containing 5 and 15 g per cent of haemoglobin before and after the addition of 10 mEq/litre of acid and 10 mEq/litre of base.

normal buffer base is subtracted from the buffer base of the sample the true excess of deficit of base will be obtained. This is equivalent to the base excess.

In practice the buffer line is determined by equilibrating two aliquots of the blood sample with two different CO_2–O_2 gas mixtures: the pH of each is then read with a glass electrode system. The pH of the third aliquot of the blood sample is then interpolated in the buffer line and the PCO_2 is read off the ordinate.

The equilibration with the known CO_2–O_2 mixtures is usually performed in the microtonometer (Fig. 12.5). This consists of two

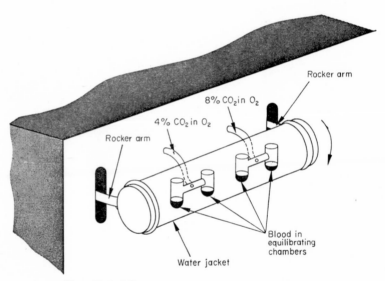

FIG. 12.5. Microtonometer on Astrup apparatus.

H-shaped glass tubes surrounded by water at 37°C. Humidified CO_2 in O_2 gas mixtures (usually 4 per cent CO_2 in the left-hand side and 8 per cent CO_2 in the right) enter the tonometer via the horizontal limb of the H and flush each of the two vertical tubes. About 0·15 ml of blood is injected into each of the four vertical tubes and the whole tonometer is then shaken at 2500 r.p.m. for 3–5 minutes. Whilst this is proceeding the pH of the original blood sample is determined in duplicate. At the conclusion of the equilibration the pH of the four blood samples is

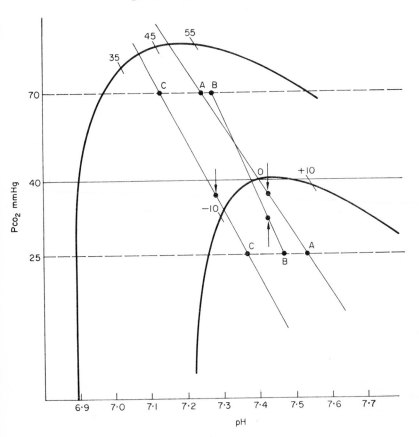

Fig. 12.6. Sources of error in the use of the Astrup technique. Line A–A represents a normal buffer line determined by the pH of the blood when equilibrated with gases of $Pco_2 = 70$ and 25 mmHg. The base excess is zero.

Points B–B represent the pH's recorded when equilibration with the gases is incomplete. If the pH of the original blood sample is now interpolated in this line the Pco_2 so determined is too low. Line C–C represents the effects of using inaccurate buffers or the presence of an abnormal liquid junction potential. Since all three blood pH readings are affected equally the Pco_2 is correct but the base estimate is in error. The error illustrated in B–B can be detected by checking whether the patient's haemoglobin corresponds to that illustrated on the buffer-base curve (see Fig. 12.7).

measured (this yields duplicates on each gas) and a $pH/\log P_{CO_2}$ plot is drawn.

The accuracy of measurement with this technique depends on a number of factors. First, it is important to determine the exact concentration of CO_2 in the 4 per cent and 8 per cent CO_2 in O_2 mixtures. The cylinders can be analysed with a Haldane apparatus or a special certificate of analysis can be obtained from the manufacturers. This gas must then be humidified by passing it through the thermostatted bubbling chambers. Then the P_{CO_2} equals per cent $CO_2 \times$ (P.B. − W.V.P. at 37°C) where P.B. = barometric pressure and W.V.P. = water vapour pressure (= 47 mmHg at 37°C).

The second important source of error arises from incomplete equilibration with the CO_2–O_2 mixtures. This type of error is increased if the patient's P_{CO_2} lies outside the range of CO_2 concentrations employed for equilibration. When equilibrating samples in the microtonometer it is important that the tonometer excursion is at least 1·4 mm so that an adequate surface of blood is exposed to the gases (Kelman, Coleman & Nunn 1966). Furthermore, the volume of blood must be restricted so that it does not spill over into the horizontal limb of the tonometer. Equilibration will be complete in 2–3 minutes if small quantities of blood are used, but with the recommended volume of 0·15 ml equilibration will not be complete in less than 4–5 minutes. This time may need to be extended if blood viscosity is increased (e.g. if the haematocrit is high). Incomplete equilibration can often be detected by inspecting the slope of the buffer line (Fig. 12.6) or by checking the haemoglobin concentration indicated on the top scale. This should agree with the true haemoglobin within ±3 g per cent. If the base excess is zero the haemoglobin concentration may be read directly off the scale by extending the buffer line to cut this scale. If, however, there is a negative or positive base excess it is necessary to determine the haemoglobin by adding or subtracting an equal number of milliequivalents from the point of intersection of the buffer line with the buffer base scale (Fig. 12.7). The greatest error in equilibration is liable to occur at the pH point which is furthest from the original blood pH, since the change in $P\text{co}_2$ during equilibration follows an approximately exponential course.

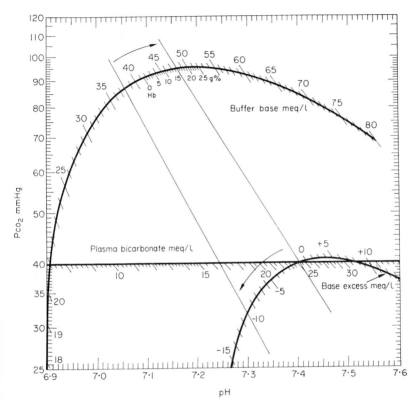

FIG. 12.7. Method of checking slope of buffer line when base excess is not zero. In this example base excess is −10 mEq/l so that 10 mEq/l must be *added* to buffer base value to obtain haemoglobin concentration (see arrows).

The third source of error is inaccuracy of the pH measurement due either to an error in measurement or failure to adjust the electrode temperature to 37°C (see page 217). With care, an accuracy of ±2 mmHg $P\text{co}_2$ and ±2·5 mEq/litre base excess can be achieved.

When interpreting the values for the non-respiratory component of acid-base balance it must be remembered that the buffer line plotted on the Siggaard–Andersen nomogram refers to *in vitro* conditions. *In vivo* the buffer line differs, because a certain amount of the bicarbonate generated by the addition of

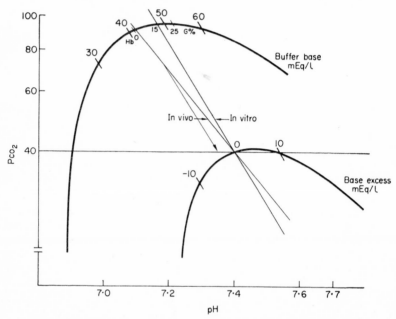

FIG. 12.8. Error in acid-base measurement due to the difference between *in vitro* and *in vivo* equilibration lines. It is assumed that the patient normally has a P_{CO_2} of 40 mmHg and base excess of zero. An acute respiratory acidosis is then induced (*in vivo curve*) and the blood sampled at a P_{CO_2} of 75 mmHg. When this blood sample is equilibrated *in vitro* the equilibration line will be displaced to the left. The apparent base deficit is indicated by the arrow.

CO_2 passes into the cells. The body as a whole, therefore, does not buffer a change in P_{CO_2} as well as blood alone, and the whole-body buffer line has a slope which is comparable with a dilute Hb solution of about 5 g per cent, i.e. the slope is more horizontal than the *in vitro* buffer line. Consequently, if a blood sample is taken from a patient with a high P_{CO_2} and then equilibrated as described above, it will appear to have a base content which is below the value which would have been obtained if the blood had been sampled when the P_{CO_2} was normal (Fig. 12.8). This error only exceeds 3–4 mEq/litre when the P_{CO_2} is above 90 mmHg, so for most practical purposes it can be ignored.

The CO_2 electrode
The electrode consists of a glass pH electrode with a flattened tip which is in contact with a thin film of sodium bicarbonate solution trapped in cellophane, Joseph paper or nylon mesh. The

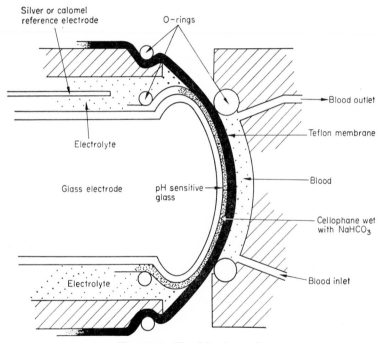

FIG. 12.9. The CO_2 electrode.

bicarbonate solution is separated from the CO_2 (in solution or in gaseous form) by a thin teflon or latex rubber membrane which is permeable to CO_2 but not to liquids or solids. CO_2 diffuses into the bicarbonate solution and the change in pH is recorded by the electrode (Fig. 12.9). To ensure accuracy to ± 1 mmHg it is essential to use a stable pH meter which can discriminate changes in pH of 0·002 pH unit. Before use the electrode must be calibrated with two known concentrations of CO_2 (such as 4 per cent and 8 per cent in O_2). A standardising gas with a Pco_2 close to that of the blood sample is then read before and after each determination. It takes about 3 minutes for the electrode to reach equilibrium with each sample of blood and gas, even if one or two increments of sample are added to speed up the response (Lunn & Mapleson 1963). The electrode is thermostatted to $37°C \pm 0·1°C$ and must be maintained exactly at this temperature to ensure stability. The cuvette must be kept filled with wash solution when not in use and the gases used for calibration must be humidified and flushed through very gently. Most CO_2 electrodes have a cuvette volume of about 0·3 ml, but usually about 1 ml of sample is required to ensure a satisfactory result. With care and patience an accuracy of ± 1 mmHg is attainable. The electrode is not affected by N_2O or O_2 and is therefore most useful for gas or blood-gas measurements during anaesthesia.

CO_2 electrodes are relatively reliable, but a small hole in the membrane can produce aberrant results with liquids even though gases read correctly. This is due to the passage of H^+ ions from the liquid into the bicarbonate solution. The membrane can be checked electrically to obviate this source of error. An alternative test is to equilibrate a dilute solution of hydrochloric acid with gas of a known Pco_2 and then to read this in the electrode. If it reads correctly it is unlikely that there is a hole in the membrane.

OXYGEN

Arterial oxygenation may be assessed by measuring the tension, saturation or content, the relationship between these three measurements being determined by the shape and position of the O_2 dissociation curve (Fig. 12.10). In the past, Po_2 was determined directly by the analysis of a gas bubble equilibrated with the blood sample. This was technically difficult, and nowadays Po_2 is usually measured directly by means of the oxygen electrode. Saturation is determined by photometric techniques involving the transmission or reflection of light at certain wavelengths, or from measurements of oxygen content and capacity by the Van Slyke apparatus:

$$O_2 \text{ saturation} = \frac{O_2 \text{ content}}{O_2 \text{ capacity}}$$

O_2 content can also be determined by driving the O_2 in the red cell into solution and measuring the change in Po_2.

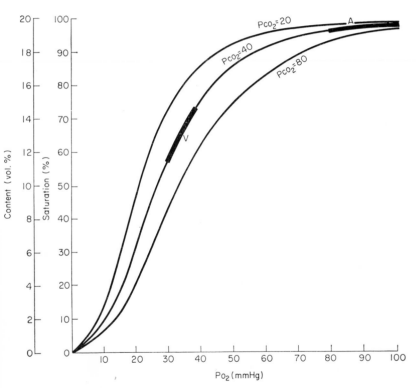

FIG. 12.10. The O_2 dissociation curve. The normal arterial (A) and venous (V) ranges are shown.

Oxygen electrode
The oxygen electrode consists of a platinum cathode and a silver anode. In most modern electrodes the cathode consists of a thin

wire of about 20 μ diameter sealed into a glass rod, whilst the anode consists of a silver wire. Both electrodes dip into a pool of electrolyte which is buffered to minimise the effect of CO_2 on the electrode. The tip of the cathode is separated from the gas or liquid in the cuvette by a plastic membrane which is permeable to gases, but not to solids or liquids (Fig. 12.11). When a polarising voltage is applied, electrons from the cathode combine with

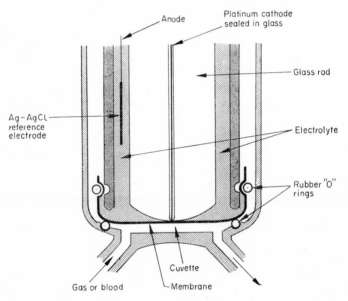

FIG. 12.11. The O_2 electrode.

O_2 molecules, reducing them to water. This is an example of a general phenomenon and there is a characteristic voltage at which any element in solution is predominantly reduced. In the case of oxygen this is 0·6 volts. In the immediate vicinity of the cathode, therefore, the oxygen tension is zero, and this creates a diffusion gradient for oxygen between the sample and the cathode. It is the movement of oxygen molecules down the diffusion gradient which enables the process of electro-reduction to proceed, and is responsible for the small current which results.

The higher the oxygen tension in the sample, the steeper the gradient, and the greater the current that is associated with the movement of the oxygen molecules. This small current which is proportional to oxygen tension is amplified and displayed as a voltage drop across a high resistance by a voltmeter. The zero point is usually set with oxygen free nitrogen. Cylinders of this gas have a black shoulder marked with a white spot. It is therefore known as 'white spot' nitrogen. The span or gain control is set with air or oxygen. A third gas is used to check the linearity of the instrument. Air is used as a calibrating gas for a Po_2 which is expected to be below 250 mmHg and oxygen if the Po_2 is expected to be higher. The calibrating gas is inserted into the cuvette before and after each measurement and the membrane is kept continually moist by frequent washings with an anti-septic–detergent wash solution. The electrode response should be complete within 30–60 seconds. As with the CO_2 electrode, careful temperature control at $37°C \pm 0.1°C$ is necessary.

In most oxygen electrodes the Po_2 reading obtained with a blood sample is less than the reading obtained with gas of the same Po_2. This blood-gas difference averages 4 per cent of the reading with the newer electrodes which use small diameter cathodes. Bigger differences were found in the larger electrodes but these could be reduced by stirring the blood during measurement. It is thought that the blood-gas difference is due to a distortion of the diffusion gradient close to the membrane, caused by the oxygen consumed by the electrode, and that greater consumption of oxygen by the larger electrodes accounted for their larger blood-gas difference. The blood-gas difference can be determined by measuring the Po_2 of blood equilibrated with gas of a known Po_2 in a tonometer (Adams & Morgan-Hughes 1967). Thirty per cent glycerine in water has a similar viscosity to a blood sample of normal haemoglobin concentration and can also be used.

In careful hands the accuracy of Po_2 measurement is ± 2 mmHg at tensions up to about 200 mmHg. Above this Po_2, accuracy rapidly falls off owing to the rapid fall in dissolved Po_2 due to metabolism by leucocytes, and to the inherent inaccuracy in the electrode and recording system. Oxygen electrodes must always be kept scrupulously clean to prevent contamination with organisms which also consume oxygen.

O_2 saturation

Although O_2 saturation can be measured *in vivo* by measuring the light transmitted or reflected by the red cells flowing through the ear lobe at certain wavelengths, it is very difficult to achieve absolute values. Most instruments are therefore designed for use with blood samples.

Reflection methods. The reflection technique is employed in the Kipp Haemoreflector and in the American Optical Company's oximeter. In the first instrument light from a polychromatic source is passed through a filter so that only light in the waveband 600–700 nm passes to the cuvette, and the reflected light is then detected with a photo-electric cell, the output from this being amplified and displayed on a scale. This instrument is affected by the haemoglobin concentration and must therefore be calibrated with fully reduced and oxygenated samples of the patient's blood. The standard deviation of the differences between readings obtained on the Haemoreflector and Van Slyke apparatus using samples with oxygen saturations varying from 40—100 per cent was 2·9 per cent saturation (Cole & Hawkins 1967). The calibration curve becomes markedly alinear below 50 per cent saturation.

The American Optical oximeter utilises light of two different wavelengths. At one wavelength (the isobestic point) the percentage absorption of fully reduced and fully oxygenated haemoglobin is equal. This gives a measure of the total haemoglobin content and is unaffected by the percentage oxygen saturation. The wavelength chosen for the other measurement is that at which the difference between the absorption curves of reduced and oxyhaemoglobin is maximal. Measurements at this wavelength therefore indicate the oxygen saturation. Since the variations in haemoglobin are automatically allowed for in this instrument it does not need individual calibration for each patient. The instrument tends to read a little high when compared to the Van Slyke apparatus and, again, inaccuracy becomes more marked below 40 per cent saturation.

Transmission oximetry. In the transmission type of oximeter the blood sample is drawn into a thin cuvette and light of two different wavelengths is passed through the blood sample, the percentage absorption being detected with a photocell. Measurements may be made on a standard spectrophotometer utilising a special thin cell or on other transmission oximeters specially designed for the task. Although the wavelengths used in different instruments vary, the principle of making two measurements, one at the isobestic point and one at another wavelength, still apply.

The principles of spectrophotometry have been dealt with more fully in Chapter 6.

The Van Slyke apparatus

Although both volumetric and manometric methods are described, most laboratories now use the manometric technique for measuring oxygen or carbon dioxide content. The apparatus consists essentially of a burette of known volume and a mercury column for measuring the pressure in the burette. A mercury reservoir is used to aspirate the reagents into the measuring chamber: it can also be used to create a vacuum in the burette (Fig. 12.12). After checking the apparatus for leaks, the chemical reagents to be used are de-gassed by shaking under reduced pressure in the burette. The gases are driven off and the reagents stored anaerobically in separate burettes. One millilitre of blood is then introduced into the Van Slyke burette with an Ostwald pipette and an acid–saponin mixture is added to haemolyse the blood and drive off all the gases. The mixture is shaken under reduced pressure and the total volume of the extracted gases is measured by recording the pressure on the manometer after the gases have been reduced to a known volume in the burette by means of the mercury reservoir. An absorbent solution is then added to the contents of the burette and the drop in pressure recorded. By using different solutions for the absorption of CO_2 and O_2 and noting the resultant drops in pressure it is possible to calculate the volumes of CO_2 and O_2 in the original blood sample.

The method is technically difficult, slow and inaccurate in the presence of anaesthetic gases. The accuracy obtainable is about

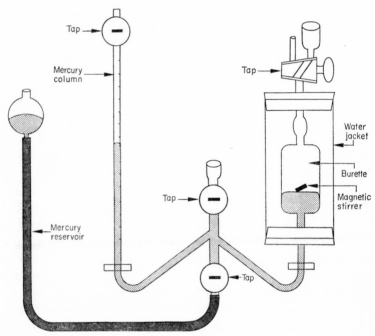

FIG. 12.12. The Van Slyke apparatus.

0·1 vol per cent for oxygen and 0·2 vol. per cent for CO_2 under the very best conditions, but it takes the average technician several months to attain this degree of competence.

MEASUREMENT OF pH

pH can be measured by the use of indicators or electrodes, and can also be calculated from a knowledge of P_{CO_2} and bicarbonate or total CO_2 content using the Henderson–Hasselbalch equation. However, as already mentioned (page 192) inaccuracies are introduced by the assumption of a fixed pK', so that the use of the Henderson–Hasselbalch equation is limited to clinical situations where there are fairly gross acid-base changes and where extreme accuracy is less important than rapidity of diagnosis. For this reason the description of the measurement of pH will be limited to the use of indicators and electrodes.

Indicators

The pH of plasma or serum can be roughly estimated by the addition of an indicator. A universal indicator can only provide an accuracy of about ±1 pH unit, but if a suitable indicator is chosen and comparison is made with the colour of the same indicator in known buffer solutions the accuracy can be increased to about ±0·2 pH units. A further increase in accuracy can be obtained by the use of more complicated instruments for measuring the absorption of transmitted light, but the techniques then become more complex and costly than those involving the use of electrodes. For this reason colorimetric techniques are now rarely used in clinical practice.

Electrodes

Although the hydrogen and quinhydrone electrodes have played an important part in research, most pH measurements are now made with the glass electrode. This is versatile, unaffected by the solution to be measured and can be used with suspensions as well as solutions. The glass electrode assembly consists of two half-cells (just as a battery consists of two half-cells) each of which develop a potential when connected together. One, the reference half-cell (commonly called the reference electrode) maintains a constant potential, whilst the other, the glass half-cell (or glass electrode), develops a potential which is proportional to the concentration of hydrogen ions present. The complete cell is shown in Fig. 12.13, and a representative commercial example in Fig. 12.14.

The potential of the calomel reference electrode is dependent solely on temperature. Since this cell reacts slowly to changes in temperature, it is important to maintain the electrodes at a constant temperature of 37°C. The calomel electrode is connected to the solution under test with a salt bridge (usually saturated or 3·5 M KCl: weaker solutions or NaCl tend to produce large liquid junction potentials). The junction between the KCl and test solution is sometimes made through a porous plug, which allows the KCl solution to flow very slowly into the test solution. In other electrodes the junction is made in a glass or plastic capillary tube, the porous plug in this arrangement usually

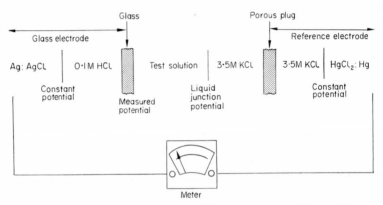

FIG. 12.13. The measurement of pH. Arrangement of electrodes and pH meter.

preventing contamination of the calomel. What matters is that there should be a sharply defined junction between the two liquids which can be formed accurately and reproducibly for each measurement, and which does not break up during the course of the measurement. The reason for this is that a potential, the liquid junction potential, is always developed at the junction between two salt solutions. Since this potential is part of the total e.m.f. of the cell, it is most important that it should remain constant during a measurement and should be reproducible with each measurement.

At 37°C the glass electrode assembly normally produces about 60 mV per pH unit change. The internal resistance of the cell is high so that if an appreciable current is drawn from the cell when the e.m.f. is measured a low value will be obtained. It is therefore essential that a meter with a high input impedance should be

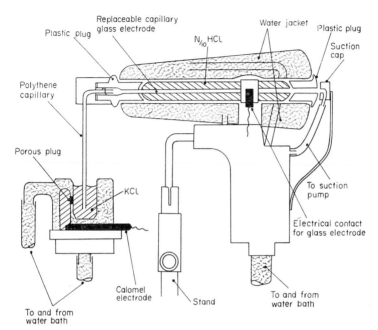

Fig. 12.14. Glass electrode assembly used in Radiometer equipment. The test solution is contained in a glass capillary which is constructed of pH sensitive glass. The column of test solution is continued into a polyethylene capillary, the end of which can be dipped into a thermostatted glass cup containing the KCl. The KCl solution in the cup can be easily renewed when contaminated. Connection to the rest of the KCl bridge and the calomel electrode is accomplished through a porous plug.

used when measuring pH. Stability and accuracy can now be obtained with high-impedance chopper or vibrating-reed amplifiers.

Buffers
Although pH has been defined as the negative logarithm of the hydrogen ion concentration, it is the activity of the hydrogen ions which affects the electrical output of the glass electrode. The

8

activity of hydrogen ions only equals the concentration of hydrogen ions in infinite dilutions. For this reason, and also because of the unknown magnitude of the liquid junction potential, it is not possible to relate the measurement of pH directly to the actual concentration of hydrogen ions present. The measurement is therefore standardised against buffer solutions. These solutions usually consist of a weak acid and its salt with a strong base, or a weak base and its salt with a strong acid. The characteristic of such a solution is that its pH remains stable despite the addition of relatively large quantities of acids or alkalis.

Unfortunately, a number of buffer scales are in use, the original Sørensen scale differing from some modern scales by as much as 0·4 pH unit. Most workers have now standardised on the National Bureau of Standards scale, since this bears the closest relation to theoretically defined values and also has a series of buffer solutions which are convenient for clinical use.

In practice, therefore, the span of the electrode is set up on phosphate buffers of pH 6·835 and 7·386, and the latter buffer is used as a reference against which blood samples are read.

Technique of pH measurement

The water bath temperature is first checked to ensure that the electrode is at $37°C \pm 0·1°C$. After setting up the electrode system so that the meter correctly spans the pH interval between the two buffers, a sample of the 7·386 buffer is placed in the electrode. The buffer adjustment is manipulated so that the needle reads exactly 7·386 on the meter, and a sample of blood is aspirated into the electrode. After a pause of 10–15 seconds (to allow diffusion of H^+ ions between the blood and the glass electrode) a second sample of blood is aspirated into the electrode. The reading is taken when the needle becomes steady, and the blood is then immediately washed out of the electrode with several aliquots of saline (water precipitates globulins which poison the glass of the electrode). Buffer is then reinserted into the electrode and the buffer reading again obtained. This should agree with the previous reading to within 0·005 pH.

Certain points of technique are important. The electrodes must be kept scrupulously clean and the KCl in the glass cup must be changed whenever it becomes contaminated. The electrode should always be kept filled with water or buffer when not in use. The sample and buffer should be introduced in two increments and care should be taken to ensure an unbroken column of fluid from one end of the capillary to the other. If the electrode response is slow the glass electrode should be filled with 0·1 per cent pepsin in $N/10$ HCl for about 30 minutes. This will dissolve the protein deposit which sometimes forms. Not infrequently the electrode responds normally with buffers but abnormally with blood samples. This error is difficult to detect, unless the electrode is checked by reading the pH of the blood sample on a second electrode system. Alternatively, the electrode may be checked with a stabilised serum preparation (G. W. Burton: see Adams, Morgan-Hughes & Sykes 1967, 1968).

TEMPERATURE CORRECTIONS

In clinical practice it is convenient to run the electrode system at 37°C and to apply correction factors to the measured Po_2, Pco_2, and pH if the patients' blood was sampled at a different temperature.

For Po_2 and Pco_2 the factors of Kelman & Nunn (1966) are usually used. For pH the correction factor suggested by Rosenthal (1948) is customarily applied. This factor is +0·0147 pH units for each 1°C fall in temperature. Burton (1965) showed that this factor depends on the original pH.

Since the significance of pH measurements at low temperatures is not clear, most clinicians correct Po_2 and Pco_2 to body temperature but measure the non-respiratory component of acid-base balance at 37°C.

BLOOD SAMPLING AND STORAGE

The samples used in blood-gas analysis may be venous, capillary or arterial. Venous samples taken with a tourniquet should never be used, since stasis markedly influences pH. Venous blood taken without stasis may be used to determine the non-respiratory component, but a correction for the arterial desaturation should be applied. 'Arterialised' venous blood obtained from the back of the hand after thorough warming of the limb may provide a useful estimate for $P\mathrm{co}_2$ and pH, but not $P\mathrm{o}_2$. Capillary blood obtained from the vasodilated ear-lobe in adults or from a heel prick in babies may also yield satisfactory results for $P\mathrm{co}_2$ and pH if the skin flow is brisk and there are no other influences, such as pain or blood-loss, which are producing vasoconstriction.

Since all these samples are subject to error and none are satisfactory for $P\mathrm{o}_2$ measurement, arterial samples are used whenever possible. Arterial blood may be sampled by intermittent puncture using a standard No. 1 (S.W.G. size 21) needle or by indwelling catheter. Catheters may be of the disposable type inserted over a needle* or may be inserted by the Seldinger (1953) technique. Catheters may be left in the radial or brachial arteries for 24–48 hours provided they are inserted carefully and are flushed with small quantities ($\frac{1}{2}$–1 ml) of heparinised saline (10 I.U./ml) at intervals of $\frac{1}{2}$–1 hour. When the needle or catheter is removed firm pressure must be applied to the site of puncture for at least 3–4 minutes. Non-occlusive pressure is then applied for a further 2–3 minutes and, if there is then no sign of haematoma formation, a firm pressure-dressing is applied.

Blood may be taken into glass or plastic syringes; $\frac{1}{2}$–1 ml of heparin is drawn into the syringe, which is held with the nozzle uppermost whilst the plunger is moved up and down. All air bubbles are now carefully expelled, only the dead space being left filled with heparin. The blood sample should be withdrawn slowly (preferably over a period of 1–2 minutes), the syringe is then capped and the blood and heparin mixed by rotating the syringe rapidly between the palms of the hands. The sample is then stored in a thermos flask containing ice and water if analysis is likely to be delayed for more than 30 minutes.

---

* 'Long-dwell' cannula (Becton-Dickinson), Angio-cath (Bard-Davol), 'Jelco' (Johnson & Johnson).

REFERENCES

ADAMS A.P. & MORGAN-HUGHES J.O. (1967) Determination of the blood-gas factor of the oxygen electrode using a new tonometer. *British Journal of Anaesthesia*, **39**, 107.

ADAMS A.P., MORGAN-HUGHES J.O. & SYKES M.K. (1967) pH and blood-gas analysis. Methods of measurement and sources of error using electrode systems. Part I. *Anaesthesia*, **22**, 575.

ADAMS A.P., MORGAN-HUGHES J.O. & SYKES M.K. (1968) pH and blood-gas analysis. Methods of measurement and sources of error using electrode systems. Part 2. *Anaesthesia*, **23**, 47.

BURTON G.W. (1965) Effects of the acid-base state upon the temperature coefficient of pH of blood. *British Journal of Anaesthesia*, **37**, 89.

CAMPBELL E.J.M. & HOWELL J.B.L. (1962) Rebreathing method for measurement of mixed venous PCO_2. *British Medical Journal*, **2**, 630.

COLE P.V. & HAWKINS L.H. (1967) The measurement of the oxygen content of whole blood. *Biomedical Engineering*, **2**, 56.

GODFREY S. (1965) Improving the reliability of the rebreathing method for measuring mixed venous PCO_2. *British Medical Journal*, **1**, 1163.

HACKNEY J.D., SEARS C.H. & COLLIER C.R. (1958) Estimation of arterial CO_2 tension by rebreathing technique. *Journal of Applied Physiology*, **12**, 425.

KELMAN G.R., COLEMAN A.J. & NUNN J.F. (1966) Evaluation of a micro-tonometer used with a capillary glass pH electrode. *Journal of Applied Physiology*, **21**, 1103.

KELMAN G.R. & NUNN J.F. (1966) Nomograms for correction of blood PO_2, PCO_2, pH and base excess for time and temperature. *Journal of Applied Physiology*, **21**, 1484.

LUNN J.N. & MAPLESON W.W. (1963) The Severinghaus PCO_2 electrode: a theoretical and experimental assessment. *British Journal of Anaesthesia*, **35**, 666.

PLESCH J. (1909) Hamodynamisch studien. *Zeitschrift für Experimentelle Pathologie und Therapie*, **6**, 380.

ROSENTHAL T.B. (1948) The effect of temperature on the pH of blood & plasma *in vitro*. *Journal of Biological Chemistry*, **173**, 25.

SELDINGER S.I. (1953) Catheter replacement of the needle in percutaneous arteriography. *Acta radiologica (Stockholm)*, **39**, 368.

SIGGAARD-ANDERSEN O. (1962) The pH-log pCO_2 blood acid-base nomogram revised. *Scandinavian Journal of Clinical and Laboratory Investigation*, **14**, 598.

SYKES M.K. (1960) Observations on a rebreathing technique for the determination of arterial PCO_2 in the apnoeic patient. *British Journal of Anaesthesia*, **32**, 256.

13

Temperature and Humidity

The increased sophistication of many surgical procedures has created a demand for accurate patient and environmental temperature control. There has also been a resurgence of interest in the potentially lethal derangements of temperature which are associated with anaesthesia. For these reasons it is important that the anaesthetist should be conversant with the instruments commonly used for measuring and controlling temperature.

Liquid or gas-expansion thermometers
This type of instrument is simple and provides a direct reading. The thermometer consists of a glass bulb, connected to an evacuated, closed capillary tube. The temperature is indicated by the position of the meniscus of a liquid such as alcohol or mercury. Providing the cross-sectional area of the capillary is constant throughout its length a linear calibration is achieved. High accuracy can be achieved but the response is somewhat slow, particularly in the clinical thermometer where there is a constriction in the stem which is designed to prevent the mercury falling until the reading has been completed.

Liquid or gas-expansion thermometers can also be made to read out on a dial by utilising the principle of the Bourdon gauge (page 90). This enables the dial to be placed remotely from the sensor. The accuracy is, however, usually much less than with a direct-reading thermometer.

Bimetallic thermometers
If strips of two metals with different coefficients of expansion are fastened together at their ends, the combined strip will bend

when heated. This principle can be used to make cheap, but not very accurate, thermometers for measuring air temperature. The bimetallic strip is used in some vaporizers to control the proportion of carrier gas flowing through the vaporizing chamber. This is accomplished by causing the strip to open or close a variable orifice.

Resistance-wire thermometers

These are based on the principle that the resistance of certain metal wires increases as their temperature increases. The metal most commonly used for this purpose is platinum, since it resists corrosion and has a large temperature coefficient of resistance. Over the range 0–100°C the change in resistance is linearly related to the change in temperature. Copper and nickel are also used. The change in resistance of the wire due to the change in temperature is usually measured by a Wheatstone bridge circuit (Chapter 3). This may be used on the null deflection principle or as a direct readout.

Platinum resistance thermometers can be made extremely accurate ($\pm0\cdot0001$°C), but the instrument then becomes somewhat fragile and slow to respond. At one time the size of the wire coil limited the application of this type of thermometer but recently much smaller probes have been produced.

Thermistor thermometers

Thermistors are semi-conductors made from fixed metallic oxides. Their resistance falls as temperature rises, but the response is non-linear. The alinearity can, however, be largely overcome by suitable circuitry. Thermistor thermometers can be made extremely sensitive ($\pm0\cdot001$°C). They are very stable, and since the probe can be made very small they have a rapid response time. This property has been utilised to monitor respiration in remote situations such as hyperbaric chambers and radiotherapy units. Although there is a very wide range of resistances available, it is difficult to match one thermistor with another and it is therefore difficult to manufacture an instrument suitable for multiple recording. Recalibration (every few months) is necessary since the thermistor tends to have an increased resistance with age.

Recently, small temperature-sensitive silicon elements have become available, their advantage being that they are readily interchangeable.

Thermocouple thermometers

If one junction formed from two dissimilar metals in an electrical circuit is heated and the other is cooled, a current will flow from one metal to the other, the current generated being proportional to the temperature gradient between the two junctions. Common combinations of metals used to make thermocouples are copper and constantan, or iron and constantan (constantan is 60 per cent copper and 40 per cent nickel). The e.m.f. generated by these junctions is relatively small so that a sensitive measuring instrument is necessary. Furthermore, it is essential to maintain the cold junction at a constant temperature or to include some compensating device which will correct for changes in ambient temperature. The latter method is used in portable instruments (Krog 1962).

The advantages of thermocouple thermometers are that they are robust and that the probes can be made in small sizes: they can therefore be made to have a quick response. In addition, the probes can be accurately reproduced so that they are very suitable for multiple recording.

Site of body-temperature measurement

Skin-temperature measurements can only be made with special probes which maintain a close application to the skin but do not in themselves affect the skin temperature.

Body temperature varies widely, depending on the site of measurement. Oesophageal temperature is thought to yield the best guide to blood temperature, but it may be reduced by hyperventilation through an endotracheal tube (Whitby & Dunkin 1968). Rectal temperature usually lags behind oesophageal temperature when body temperature is rapidly changed by surface cooling or warming, or by extracorporeal circulation.

Accurate measurements can only be made if the rectum is empty. They then provide a useful guide to 'core' temperature. When rectal temperature approaches oesophageal after rapid cooling or warming it is unlikely that a further change in temperature will occur. Nasopharyngeal temperature or the temperature of the tympanic membrane in the external auditory meatus has been used as an indication of brain temperature. However, because of the large temperature gradients which exist during rapid cooling or warming, it is unwise to assume that any temperature measurement in one part of the body reflects that existing elsewhere.

THERMOGRAPHY

The human skin behaves almost exactly as a black body radiator. This means it emits infra-red radiation with a predictable spectrum. The shortest wavelength emitted is about 3 μm, and the range extends up to several hundred micrometres. The emitted energy increases at all wavelengths as the temperature rises, and if a narrow range of frequencies can be detected, the amount of radiant emission is proportional to temperature.

Detectors are of two basic kinds: temperature-sensitive devices such as thermistors and thermocouples, or photon-sensitive devices. The former have a high sensitivity but the response time is slow. They are thus suitable for measuring the temperatures of a small or uniform area whose temperature is not changing quickly. They are unsuitable for use in scanning cameras. Filters are used to minimise the effects of other wavelengths, such as reflected sunlight, and the elements are shielded from ambient temperatures. For heat scans the most versatile photon-sensitive material is indium antimonide, which is a photo-conductive material which produces a small current when infra-red radiation between 1 μm and 6 μm impinges on it. The detector has to be kept very cold in liquid nitrogen to eliminate thermal noise arising in the detector itself.

The field is scanned, rather like a television picture, successively, both vertically and horizontally. The speed of response

8*

is such that as many as a hundred individual points in a frame can be scanned four times a second. The information can be displayed on a cathode-ray oscilloscope, intensity modulated, so that hotter areas appear brighter.

The main fields of application of thermographic scanning have been in the diagnosis of breast tumours, the location of deep perforating varicose veins of the leg, the site of vascular occlusions, and the location of the placenta. No direct applications to anaesthesia have yet been reported, but the measurement of changes in blood flow is an obvious possibility, particularly in an intensive care situation.

MEASUREMENT OF HUMIDITY

There are two situations in anaesthetic practice in which the control of humidity is of the utmost importance. The first is in the operating theatre where a high relative humidity is maintained to decrease the risk of static sparks. The other situation arises when a patient breathes through an endotracheal or tracheostomy tube and extra humidity must be provided to prevent crusting of secretions.

Two measures of humidity are in common use.

Absolute humidity is the actual amount of water vapour contained in a given volume of gas at a given temperature and pressure. It is expressed in grams of water vapour per cubic metre of gas.

Relative humidity is the actual amount of water vapour present in the gas expressed as a percentage of the amount that the same volume of gas would contain at the same temperature and pressure if it were fully saturated.

The amount of water vapour required to saturate a given volume of air increases with temperature (Fig. 13.1). Consequently, air which is fully saturated at 20°C will be only about 30 per cent saturated when warmed to 37°C. Normally the additional moisture required to saturate the inspired air is added during its passage through the nose, mouth and trachea. However, if the upper respiratory tract is bypassed by an endotracheal or tracheostomy tube it is necessary either to warm the air to 37°C and fully saturate it before entry to the trachea or to add droplets of water which will vaporize and saturate the air when it is warmed to 37°C in the body.

Measurements of humidity are made by instruments termed hygrometers.

Regnault's hygrometer. A silver tube is cooled gradually by the evaporation of liquid ether. When the tube cools to the dewpoint

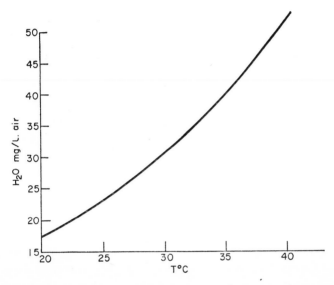

FIG. 13.1. Water content of fully saturated air at various temperatures.

of the surrounding air (i.e. the point at which the air becomes fully saturated), small droplets of water will condense on the outside of the silver tube. If the temperature of the ether is now measured the absolute humidity can be read from the graph (Fig. 13.1) or from tables.

Hair hygrometer. A human hair increases in length as the humidity of the surrounding air increases. If one end of the hair is fixed and the other is attached to a light lever system which magnifies the change in length, the scale can be suitably calibrated and a direct reading of relative humidity obtained. The range is limited to 15–85 per cent relative humidity and the accuracy is not high.

Wet and dry bulb thermometer. Two mercury-in-glass thermometers are mounted side by side. The bulb of one is exposed to the air whilst the bulb of the other is surrounded by a small wick which dips into a water reservoir. The temperature of the wet bulb depends on the rate of evaporation, and hence on the humidity of the surrounding air, and is therefore lower than the temperature of the dry bulb. As humidity is increased the rate of evaporation becomes less and the temperature difference between the two bulbs decreases. The relative humidity is determined from tables which relate the dry and wet bulb temperatures to the humidity.

Humidity transducers. These utilise the change in electrical characteristics which occurs in a substance when it absorbs water. The substance is usually used as a resistor or as the dielectric portion of a capacitor, and the change in resistance or capacitance is detected by an electronic circuit. Such an instrument can be made extremely sensitive and can be used as part of a servo-system to control humidity in air-conditioning systems.

Weighing. When water droplets are present in the air the absolute humidity may exceed the value for saturated air at that temperature. The measurement of humidity can then only be accomplished by either warming the air so that all the droplets are evaporated or by condensing the water vapour and weighing the quantity of water in a known volume of air. Allowance must then be made for the water vapour still present in the saturated vapour over the condensed water. An alternative technique is to absorb the water vapour in concentrated sulphuric acid, silica gel or anhydrous calcium chloride and again to determine the quantity present by weighing. If these methods are used the air must be passed through a number of chambers arranged in series, so that the completeness of absorption can be checked. (There should be no weight gain in the terminal chamber.)

Mass spectrometer. This instrument (see page 184) can be used to measure the water vapour pressure (Hayes & Robinson

1969). However, the expense of such an instrument precludes its general use.

REFERENCES

HAYES B. & ROBINSON J.S. (1970) An assessment of methods of humidification of inspired gas. *British Journal of Anaesthesia*, **42**, 94.

KROG I. (1962) Electrical measurements of body temperature. In: *Electrical Measurements in Anaesthesiology* (ed. H. Poulsen). Acta Anaesthesiologica Scandinavica, Suppl. XI.

WHITBY J.D. & DUNKIN L.J. (1968) Temperature differences in the oesophagus: preliminary study. *British Journal of Anaesthesia*, **40**, 991.

FURTHER READING

ROBERTSON T.L. (1968) Clinical temperature measurement-survey. *Biomedical and Scientific Instruments*, **4**, 303.

14

Biological Potentials

The electrical activity which accompanies changes in cell membrane permeability can be detected from most of the surface of the body, as well as from electrodes placed in close proximity to specialized tissues.

In routine monitoring, the electrocardiogram (E.C.G.) is the most common potential which is detected and displayed, whilst the electroencephalogram (E.E.G.) may be important in a few situations. The electrical activity recorded from muscles (the electromyogram, or E.M.G.) is useful in the differential diagnosis of muscle diseases and neuromuscular transmission defects. Despite the obvious application in anaesthesia, such recordings, whether from surface electrodes, electrodes within muscle fibres or specially located at the end-plate, have remained within the field of research, and clinical management depends on the assessment of the power developed in a muscle in response to various forms of electrical stimulation of the motor nerve. The technique of recording changes in the electrical impedance of tissues has been applied to measurements of respiration, cardiac output, limb blood flow, the effects of sedation, and the level of autonomic activity. All these applications have certain instrumental problems in common, although the relative importance of each problem varies with the application. Before considering the applications separately, it will be convenient to discuss the general problems associated with the recording of biological potentials.

INTERFERENCE

As was pointed out in Chapter 1, the first essential in any instrumentation system is that the signal/noise ratio should be high. Noise may originate in the patient or his surroundings and

228

in the instruments used for recording, amplification and display. Instrumental noise can be reduced by careful design, the use of high grade components and adequate screening. However, noise arising from the patient or his surroundings is often more difficult to eradicate.

Noise originating from the patient
The electrical changes associated with the heart beat produce potential differences of about 0·5–2 mV on the surface of the body, whilst the E.E.G. signal on the scalp has a magnitude of about 50 μV. The E.C.G. signal may thus distort the E.E.G. signal, whilst both these signals may be submerged by the much larger potentials produced by muscular movement. The choice of electrode and electrode site is important, and the use of amplifiers with high powers of discrimination may prove invaluable. For example, although the E.C.G. signal is much larger than the E.E.G. it is rarely a troublesome source of interference, since the E.C.G. potentials are substantially in phase at all points on the head and can therefore be eliminated by using an amplifier with a high in-phase rejection ratio (see p. 232). Muscle interference has a much higher frequency than the components of an E.E.G. and can often be eliminated by cutting the high-frequency response of the amplifier to a level which does not interfere greatly with the characteristics of the E.E.G.

Noise originating from sources outside the patient
Interference from outside sources is due principally to electrostatic or electromagnetic induction.
   Electrostatic induction. When a charged body is brought close to an uncharged one it will induce an equal and opposite charge in the uncharged body. In a similar manner, if a mains cable lies close to a patient or to an input lead to an amplifier it will induce a charge in the patient or lead. This charge will vary with the potential to which the mains lead is exposed and will therefore alternate at mains frequency. Figure 14.1 indicates the situation which develops when a patient is near a mains cable. The patient

acts as one plate of a capacitor whilst the mains lead constitutes the other plate. The patient also acts as a capacitance with respect to earth. Since the mains lead is also connected to earth,

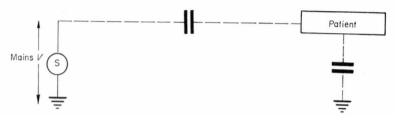

Fig. 14.1. Electrostatic induction in a patient, due to a mains lead. S = source of alternating current.

there is an effective a.c. circuit which will conduct an alternating current through the patient even though there is no direct connection between the patient and the mains. Furthermore, it should be noted that the current in the patient is induced solely

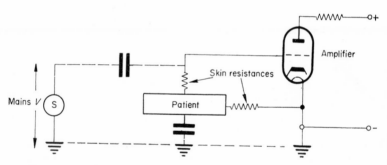

Fig. 14.2. Electrostatic induction in a wire leading from the patient to an amplifier.

by the changes in *potential* in the mains lead: there is no need for a current to flow through the wire. This type of interference may therefore occur when all the other apparatus in the room is switched off. Figure 14.2 shows the effects of electrostatic induction in the wire leading from the patient to the amplifier. In this case the lead acts as one plate of a capacitor and the induced charge in the lead is therefore superimposed on the signal from the patient. The voltage which appears in the lead depends on the resistance associated with the leads and patient, on the magnitude of the mains voltage and on the proximity of the mains cable. The induced voltage is minimised by minimising the resistance of the patient–lead combination and by increasing the distance between the lead and mains cable.

Electromagnetic induction. This form of interference occurs in the vicinity of wires carrying alternating currents. When a current is flowing it generates a magnetic field, and there are thus alternating magnetic fields around and through the patient

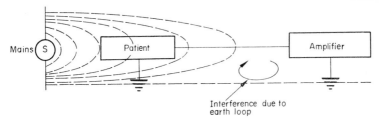

Fig. 14.3. The effects of multiple earths.

and any connections leading to other apparatus. When a magnetic field decays or builds up, any lines of force which cut a loop of wire lying within the field induce a voltage in the loop, the magnitude of the voltage depending on the strength of current in the wire carrying the alternating current and the size of the loop (see Chapter 3). Now, the individual leads each form a loop which incorporates both the patient and the apparatus. If, therefore, unequal e.m.f.'s are induced in the various loops, a.c. interference will occur. To minimise this type of interference all the leads should be kept close together, and twisted around one another as much as possible.

Another common cause of magnetically coupled interference is multiple earthing of the patient (see Fig. 14.3). If the recording apparatus is earthed, and the patient is separately earthed, for example, by the diathermy pad, a large loop is made through earth. An alternating voltage is induced in this *earth loop* by alternating mains currents. It may be necessary to disconnect the earth connection on the apparatus to cure this form of interference. (It is *not* correct to disconnect the diathermy earth!)

Elimination of a.c. interference

There are two methods of eliminating a.c. interference: discrimination and screening.

Discrimination. It has been pointed out that the electrostatically or electromagnetically induced voltages in the patient or lead are cyclical and in phase with the a.c. mains. Furthermore, these voltages appear almost simultaneously at all points on the patient. If two leads are attached to the patient at different points they will therefore record a difference in potential due to the biological signal plus the cyclical changes in potential due to the induced voltage. By using a *balanced amplifier* or a *balanced input transformer* it is possible to discriminate between the 'in-phase' and 'out-of-phase' signals so that only the signals which are out of phase get through. A good balanced amplifier may have a discrimination factor of 10,000, that is to say the ratio of the amplifier gain for anti-phase (out of phase) signals to the gain for in-phase signals is 10,000 to 1. This is also called the *in-phase rejection ratio*. It should be remembered that the discrimination of an amplifier may fall considerably if the resistance of the electrodes is high.

It will be apparent that it is absolutely imperative for two input leads to be connected between the patient and the apparatus. If one lead becomes disconnected, the voltages appearing across the remaining lead are now unbalanced and 'out of phase' and the true signal is immediately swamped in a large 50 Hz waveform. So-called unipolar leads are bipolar connections, with the active lead compared with an indifferent lead connected to a point on the body which is remote from the signal, or alternatively, compared with an average signal derived from all the other leads connected together.

Screening. The type of screening required depends on the type of interference. Electrostatic screening is accomplished by placing an earthed conductor round the patient or input lead. Screening of the patient is only required in the most rigorous applications, and is rarely used in clinical practice. Screening of the leads and amplifier is, however, essential, both in laboratory and clinical situations. The screen round a lead must be connected to earth through a low resistance connection. It then acts as one plate of a capacitor, and any voltages which are induced in it are short circuited immediately to earth (Fig. 14.4). The screen and lead also function as two plates of a capacitor, but since a charge cannot build up on the screen (because it is connected to earth) there is no induced voltage in the lead.

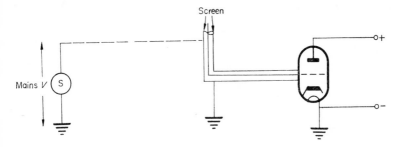

Fig. 14.4. Screening patient connections.

Screening against electromagnetic interference is more complicated. There are two approaches. In one, the lines of magnetic force are concentrated in a material of high permeability (iron or an alloy such as mu-metal) which surrounds the amplifier. Since the field is concentrated in the material the field inside is weakened. In the second approach the apparatus is enclosed in a box made of a good conductor such as copper. The magnetic field induces eddy currents in the copper and these in turn set up their own magnetic fields which tend to cancel the induced field. A similar principle is used to minimise interference in cables. By placing the wires close together and parallel to each other (e.g. twisted flex) the fields which are induced are made equal and opposite and so cancel each other out.

Other sources of interference

Interference may enter the amplifier through the mains, and for this reason most biological amplifiers are provided with a carefully filtered and smoothed high-tension supply. Outside interference also arises from surgical diathermy, sparking of switch or motor commutator contacts and other electrical equipment. Broadcast radio is seldom strong enough to provide a serious source of interference, but has caused trouble on occasions.

REQUIREMENTS OF BIOLOGICAL AMPLIFIERS

One essential requirement which has already been discussed above, is a high in-phase rejection ratio. Another important

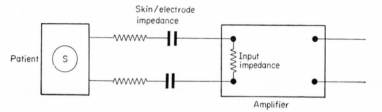

FIG. 14.5. The effect of amplifier input impedance and skin resistance on the recording of biological potentials.

property of amplifiers is their input impedance, that is the total resistance to alternating currents (see Chapter 3). It will be recalled that impedance comprises both resistance and reactance, and reactances may be either inductive or capacitative. If one considers the body as a generator of alternating e.m.f.'s, one can view the amplifier as part of an external circuit and in series with the impedance of the skin and electrodes (see Fig. 14.5). The impedance of the skin is largely resistive and the reactive component is mainly capacitative. If a current flows in this external circuit, the signal at the amplifier input is attenuated across the skin–electrode resistance. This attenuation is least when the input impedance of the amplifier is high when compared with skin resistance. For E.E.G. work, in which the signal voltage and the electrode impedances are both small, amplifier input impedances need to be of the order of 10,000,000 ohms (10 MΩ). For E.M.G. and E.C.G. amplification, input impedances may be smaller, but still in the megohm range.

The band-width (see Chapter 3) of the amplifier must cover the range of frequencies that are of importance in the signal. The American Heart Association standard for E.C.G. machines (1967) specifies a flat response from 0·14 Hz up to 50 Hz and allows up to 30 dB attenuation at 0·05 Hz and 100 Hz (30 dB is a 1000-fold loss). E.E.G.'s can be recorded satisfactorily using an amplifier with more voltage amplification, and a similar band-width, although purpose-built machines usually have a band-width that extends from 0·5 Hz up to nearly 100 Hz. E.M.G.'s, or nerve action potential recordings, require a flat response from about 20 Hz up to at least 1 kHz, and preferably up to 10 kHz, to record the high frequencies contained in the signal.

Biological amplifiers need to have relatively long time constants (see Chapter 3). This is because the resistance of the skin–electrode junction can vary very considerably, and develop slowly changing (d.c.) voltages which, if amplified, would drive the trace right off the recorder. The time constant of an E.C.G. amplifier is fixed, and is usually 3 seconds, which means that the trace will return to within 95 per cent of its base line position in 9 seconds, after being displaced by a d.c. voltage. E.E.G. machines provide a selection of time constants of 0·03, 0·1, 0·3 and 1 second. The selection of a very short time-constant will result in the attenuation of the low frequency components of the recording.

Filters are usually incorporated, to introduce additional attenuation at one or other end of the frequency range. For example, a high-frequency filter may be necessary to 'clean up' an E.E.G. trace when there are muscle artefacts.

Calibration voltages may be incorporated so that the gain of the amplifiers can be correctly adjusted. It is customary to calibrate the E.C.G. so that a 1 mV input will produce a 1 cm deflection of the trace, and the E.E.G. so that 100 μV (0·1 mV) produces this deflection.

ELECTRODES

The importance of having an amplifier input impedance significantly greater than the electrode–skin resistance has already been mentioned. At one time, biological signals could only be displayed using string galvanometers, and since these inevitably had a low input impedance, it was vital to lower the electrode–skin resistance as much as possible. This was achieved by using an electrode with a large area, applying electrically conductive jelly, and abrading away the cornified layer of the skin in which the major part of the skin resistance resides. With the introduction of the valve amplifier, very high input impedances were easily obtained, rendering much electrode mystique pointless. With amplifiers having input impedances of over 2 MΩ it has been shown that perfectly satisfactory traces can be obtained using K–Y jelly, mustard, tomato ketchup, handcream, toothpaste, or even with no jelly at all (Lewes 1965). A further advantage is that electrodes with much smaller areas of contact can be used, although there has perhaps been a tendency to move too far in this direction without appreciating the consequences. For instance, subcutaneous needles have an appreciable impedance which, being largely capacitative, is marked at low frequencies. This gives rise to spurious features in the E.C.G., particularly diphasic T-waves and increased S-waves. It may also give the appearance of S–T depression. This fact is now of increasing importance, because transistorized amplifiers have a lower input impedance than valve amplifiers, and an unduly high electrode resistance will more readily lead to the production of this artefact (Meyer 1967).

A high electrode–skin resistance has another undesirable consequence, in that it markedly accentuates the magnitude of capacitatively-coupled a.c. interference. If fine bore concentric needle electrodes are used for electromyography, it may be necessary to screen not only the apparatus but also the patient.

The nature of the electrode is also of importance. When two dissimilar metals are in contact via an electrolyte solution, the one which is the more electropositive reacts with the electrolyte giving off positive ions, and so becomes negatively charged. These ions migrate to the other metal and give it a positive charge. When a current flows between the two metals, a neutral layer is deposited on the positive plate, which increases its resistance. This process is known as *polarisation*. The least electropositive conductor is carbon, and those metals which are nearest to it in the electrochemical scale are least prone to this effect. These are platinum and silver. Polarisation effects are least at high frequencies, and distortion is chiefly due to attenuation of lower frequencies. The smaller the e.m.f.'s being recorded, the more vital it becomes to use non-polarising electrodes. Electrodes of silver, coated with silver chloride, or platinum, are essential for good quality E.E.G. recordings. Stainless steel is less satisfactory, but is adequate as a surface electrode for E.C.G. and E.M.G. signals. Needle electrodes have a small surface area in contact with the patient, and consequently have a high impedance. Concentric stainless-steel needles have a particularly high impedance, and if their use is imperative, a high-input impedance amplifier is essential unless an element of trace distortion is acceptable.

Signal display

Galvanometer pens are satisfactory for E.C.G. and E.E.G. trace display; a hot stylus on pre-treated paper, or ink jets, are both common methods. E.M.G. traces are usually displayed on an oscilloscope which can be photographed if required, or traced directly onto light-sensitive paper. Mechanically linked recorders do not possess a high enough frequency response for E.M.G. traces.

Safety

There is potentially a greater risk to the patient in recording biological potentials than in almost any other form of measurement. This is because there is a deliberate connection between the patient and apparatus containing sources of high voltages. There is, therefore, a need for the utmost care in biological potential recording. Transcardiac currents of only a few milliamps can cause ventricular fibrillation, and low-current fuses should be incorporated in the leads to the patient, or the input isolated from the rest of the apparatus by appropriate circuitry. This is particularly important when cardiac catheters are in position, since these bypass the normal skin and electrode impedances, and provide a direct electrical path to the heart (Hopps & Roy 1963). Fatalities have occurred when monitoring apparatus was being connected to a patient who was already connected to other electrical apparatus and faulty earthing or incorrect polarity allowed unexpected currents to flow. It is important to monitor the pulse or E.C.G. while electrical connections are being made.

TISSUE IMPEDANCE MEASUREMENT

The impedance of tissues depends on their constitution. When a small alternating current is applied across a portion of tissue, changes in its impedance can be detected as a change of a.c. voltage between the electrodes. Changes in impedance occur when the average composition of the tissue between the electrodes changes. This can occur, for example, in a limb which, because of vasodilatation, contains a greater amount of blood, or across the thorax when the intake of air causes a change in thoracic geometry.

Absolute calibration, based on the actual values of impedance, is virtually impossible. So much depends on the position of the electrodes, the frequency of current employed, and the tissue structure of the individual. However, changes in impedance can often be shown to have a reasonably linear approximation to the function under examination, and the voltage changes can thus be calibrated empirically in an individual case.

The frequencies employed in impedance measurements are high enough to prevent polarisation of the electrodes; for impedance spirometry frequencies of tens to hundreds of kHz are employed.

For impedance spirometry the electrodes are placed on either side of the chest in the mid-axillary line, and the gain is adjusted to give an adequate change of signal during the respiratory cycle.

If a semi-quantitative display is the only requirement, this is sufficient. For calibration, however, the actual impedance of the patient at end-expiration is determined by substituting a variable known resistance between the electrodes. Since the changes in impedance are mainly resistive, a non-inductive resistance is used. The calibrating resistance is then altered in known steps, and the change in signal noted. This gives ΔZ, the change in impedance, and this must now be related to ΔV, the change in volume which produces the same voltage change when the patient is connected. This can be done by allowing the patient to breathe in and out of a spirometer, or if paralysed, by inflating with a known volume. If $\Delta Z/\Delta V$ is approximately linear, any change in impedance can be calibrated in terms of volume (Baker & Hill 1969). These authors have also published a circuit diagram of a suitable apparatus (Hill & Baker 1969).

There is no inherent reason why the same technique, with differently placed electrodes should not be able to demonstrate the change in size of the heart with each heart beat.

In impedance plethysmography of a limb it is possible to calibrate roughly by the use of simultaneous venous occlusion or strain gauge plethysmography. However, if such a method is readily available, there is no need for the less accurate impedance measurements. Consequently, impedance measurements are employed when the actual values are not of interest and only changes in a state of varying magnitude are required. Thus the technique has been used as an objective indication of anxiety, which affects limb blood flow, and for monitoring ventilation.

ELECTRICAL STIMULATORS

It is sometimes desired to reverse the process of recording biological potentials and to apply an electric current to an excitable tissue. This may be done by electrodes applied directly to a nerve or within the substance of a muscle, or by electrodes applied to the skin. Large currents are also applied to the heart, or across the chest wall for purposes of arresting arrhythmias and inducing a refractory pause, and also for applying the stimulus to initiate the cardiac contraction. The technology of cardiac pacemakers has been covered by Siddons & Sowton (1967), and the problems encountered in clinical anaesthesia have been reviewed by Scott (1970), and will not be discussed further.

Clinical nerve stimulators

There are several portable nerve stimulators available on the market for clinical use. The variables in the design of a nerve stimulator are the voltage of the stimulus, the duration of the stimulus and the shape of the waveform of the stimulus. The wave form is most frequently a square wave, which is relatively easy to produce. The voltage may be varied by a rheostat, and the range of voltages available depends on the intended use. Much higher voltages are necessary for instruments in which the voltage is to be applied to the intact skin, than in those which are applied by needle electrodes to the nerve. Some machines have a range of voltages to allow for either type of usage. There is a critical duration of stimulus, around 5 milliseconds, below which the current will not cause sufficient depolarization of the nerve to initiate a propagated impulse. It is also undesirable to apply a current for too long, since this may initiate a train of impulses. The duration of the stimulus, in fact, should be shorter than the refractory period. This is quite short for a nerve which may conduct impulses at rates approaching a 100 or more per second.

In the differential diagnosis of neuromuscular disorders, it is frequently desired to observe the effects of a single stimulus and the effects of a fast burst of stimuli sufficient to produce a tetanic contraction of the muscle. Simple clinical instruments rarely incorporate a rate control and are usually content with a two position arrangement of slow (up to three impulses per second) and tetanic (around fifty per second) rates. However, care is necessary when interpreting the results of stimulation with some of these instruments, since the pattern of stimulus may differ from that produced by the standard laboratory stimulator (Epstein *et al.*, 1969).

Since skin resistance is a very variable quantity, it is desirable to start with the voltage control turned well down and then to increase the voltage until a satisfactory effect is produced. The efficiency of the stimulator can often be much improved by lowering the skin resistance with abrasive and conductive jelly: it is also much affected by the proximity of the electrodes to the nerve. For this reason, quantitative interpretations of the amount of current or voltage necessary to induce an impulse are quite valueless with skin electrodes.

RATEMETERS AND WARNING SYSTEMS

When a satisfactory signal has been isolated from the other electrical activity present in the body it may be processed in a number of different ways. Impulses arising from muscle or nerve are often displayed on an oscilloscope: the trace can then be photographed if a permanent record is required. The correct location of the tip of electrodes used for this kind of work is often greatly facilitated if the impulses are channelled to a loudspeaker, since this allows the pattern of discharge to be easily recognised by ear. Another way of recording the frequency with which impulses are occurring is to display the count in the form of a frequency histogram. This is accomplished by counting the number of impulses in successive time intervals: each of these counts is then displayed sequentially on a recorder.

If a signal is occurring at regular intervals (e.g. E.C.G.) it is possible to measure the rate. This may be displayed digitally or on a meter, either as the time necessary to record a fixed number of beats or as the number of beats in a fixed time interval. Usually rate is counted by causing the R-wave to trigger the meter, but the peak of the arterial pressure wave may be used equally well. Ratemeters commonly employ an integrating circuit with an R–C network. The capacitor is charged at regular intervals by the pulse from the E.C.G. and the charge is allowed to drain away through the resistance. By suitably adjusting the time constant of the system (by adjusting R and C) it is possible to arrange that the charge on the capacitor is proportional to the frequency of impulses. The charge can then be displayed on a meter.

A display of this kind lends itself to a further modification which causes a warning signal to be produced when the rate exceeds or falls below predetermined limits. Needless to say the success of such a warning system is entirely dependent on the continuity of electrode contact and the elimination of all interference. Unfortunately, the difficulty of achieving these conditions in clinical practice greatly reduces the usefulness of these systems.

Further developments in warning systems may eventually come from the use of computers to analyse pulse irregularities, for there is a suggestion that certain types of irregularity may commonly precede the onset of ventricular fibrillation. Certainly, it is now clear that the careful monitoring and treatment of arrhythmias greatly reduces the incidence of cardiac arrest in myocardial infarction.

REFERENCES

BAKER L.E. & Hill D.W. (1969) The use of electrical impedance techniques for the monitoring of respiratory pattern during anaesthesia. *British Journal of Anaesthesia*, **41**, 2.

EPSTEIN R.A., WYTE S.R., JACKSON S.H. & SITTER S. (1969) The electromechanical response to stimulation by the Block-aid Monitor. *Anesthesiology*, **30**, 43.

HILL D.W. & BAKER L.E. (1969) Impedance pneumograph. *British Journal of Anaesthesia*, **41**, 794.

HOPPS J.A. & ROY O.Z. (1963) Electrical hazards in cardiac diagnosis and treatment. *Medical Electronics & Biological Engineering* **1**, 133.

LEWES D. (1965) Electrode jelly in electrocardiography. *British Heart Journal*, **27**, 105.

MEYER J.L. (1967) Some instrument-induced errors in the E.C.G. *Journal of the American Medical Association*, **201**, 351.

Report of a committee on electrocardiography. American Heart Association (1967). *Circulation*, **35**, 583.

SCOTT D.H. (1970) Cardiac pacemakers as an anaesthetic problem. *Anaesthesia*, **25**, 87.

SIDDONS H. & SOWTON E. (1967). *Cardiac Pacemakers*. C.C. Thomas, Springfield, Illinois.

15
Measurement of Subjective Responses

Although anaesthetists are primarily concerned with ensuring the absence of pain, they are also very much concerned with the patient's feelings. In this respect, their interest in the patient as a sentient being has overlapped with psychiatry. It is probably the most difficult area of research in which to obtain meaningful and reproducible measurements.

As far as instrumentation is concerned, there are two broad aspects to consider; the production of a graded and measurable stimulus, and the measurement of objective parameters which are believed to parallel subjective experience.

Graded stimuli

The assessment of analgesic drugs has followed three main lines. One has been to use the 'natural' pain of operations as the stimulus, and to record the patient's subjective response to therapy. This assessment has sometimes been supplemented with the observers' opinions. There are a number of difficulties inherent in this approach, in particular the difficulty of producing a satisfactory scoring system and handling the resulting score statistically. However, as far as the assessment of narcotic analgesics is concerned, it seems likely that this approach may yield much more useful data than methods involving the use of artificial pain. Since this type of measurement does not fall within the ambit of this book and has been fully covered by Beecher (1959), it will not be discussed further.

Because the pain of abdominal incisions inhibits ventilation, pain relief can be assessed by measuring the improvement in respiratory function which follows its successful alleviation. Tidal volume may be reduced to a third or half the normal value on the first and second post-operative days after an upper abdominal operation, but vital capacity is often reduced to one-fifth of the normal value. The peak expiratory flow rate is also reduced. The change in vital capacity and peak flow rate resulting from the administration of analgesic drugs or the use of other methods of pain relief may be conveniently recorded with a fast spirometer or by the use of the Wright respirometer and peak flowmeter (see Chapters 9 and 10). Although these measurements yield figures which can be submitted to statistical analysis, it must be remembered that they still partly depend upon the degree of co-operation, and indeed will-power, of the subject, both of which may be modified by the sedative or other qualities of the drug in question.

Another much used investigative tool has been graded artificial pain. This allows one to measure a 'pain threshold' and to observe any modification of the threshold by drugs. An 'ideal' method for producing painful stimuli should approach the following characteristics. There should be no tissue damage at the pain threshold; the same stimulus should give a reproducible and quantifiable response under standard conditions; the stimulus should be easily applicable, and give a clear pain end-point; the stimulus should be sensitive enough to detect low analgesic activity; it should be able to differentiate between different doses of analgesic; it should be applicable in man and experimental animals. It is fair to say that no method meets this ideal. There are four groups of methods which have been used to produce experimental pain; thermal, mechanical, electrical and chemical.

The most usual form of thermal stimulus is the heat and light from a 500 or 1000 watt lamp focused on a small area of blackened skin for a fixed, short time, usually 3 seconds. The current is increased until the subject feels the sensation of pain just at the end of the exposure. One minute is allowed between exposures. For really accurate work it is necessary to control or correct for the skin temperature. An alternative approach is to keep the intensity of light constant, and vary the time of exposure. This has also been applied to the rat tail-flick test. Here the heat is focused on the rat tail, which is lying in a groove. The time taken before the tail flicks away is recorded. This, of course, is really a reflex reaction threshold, and is not necessarily comparable with the pain threshold verbally reported in man.

Although it is possible to quantify the threshold in terms of the power output of the lamp, there is no entirely satisfactory way of handling the data, particularly when it comes to assaying an analgesic. A common solution is to measure the maximum percentage increase of threshold over pre-treatment value, and plot this figure for each dose on a log/dose scale. A sigmoid curve may result. The slope of the flat part of the curve may then be used for further statistical manipulation. It would be fair to say that some violence often has to be applied to the data to make them tractable.

Mechanical methods of pain production were first introduced by von Frey in 1897, who impressed horse hairs into the epidermis with a weighted balance. Gross pressure over sub-cutaneous bones, such as the shin, has been much in vogue in recent years. If the area submitted to the stimulus is controlled, the pressure, and therefore the force, can be gradually increased until pain is produced. If the increase in pressure occurs at a constant rate and the device is calibrated with an arbitrary scale of pressure units, it is possible to obtain quite reproducible values for the pressures needed to produce the sensation of pain in any individual provided that the investigator has acquired con-siderable experience in its use. It is, however, possible for the investigator to influence the result. Not all parts of the skin, for example, are equally sensitive and an area which has once been compressed may be more sensitive for a period of time thereafter. Double-blind methods are definitely desirable. Dundee & Moore (1960) have a further discussion of this method, using a spring-balance to produce the pressure.

Electrical pain is still assumed by many to be a useful and reliable tool. The most common technique utilises a measurement of the current necessary to produce pain by stimulating the tooth pulp through the dentine. There is no doubt that quite sharp, reproducible end-points can be obtained, and the sensation of pain is undeniable. However, many workers have found it to be highly inconsistent at times, and furthermore, have failed to demonstrate any change of threshold after the administration of quite acceptable analgesics. In one study, 0·5 mg of adrenaline was found to have four times the analgesic potency of 16 mg of morphine, which is hard to reconcile with usual clinical experience. The method, however, is undoubtedly more reliable in dogs.

Chemical pain is best produced by ischaemic muscle during exercise. It is necessary to standardise the force of isometric contractions and also the frequency of contractions. Under these conditions pain is felt after a constant time. It is of interest that this is the only form of artificial pain with which it has been possible to detect significant threshold changes following mild analgesics, such as aspirin, in well-controlled studies. It has also been successfully used to compare the relative analgesic potency of narcotic analgesics (Hewer & Keele 1948).

The production of a graded stimulus does not by any means solve the problem of measuring a pain threshold. At least two separate thresholds can be determined in co-operative individuals, the point at which the changing stimulus is recognised as pain, and a later time when it cannot be tolerated. It is the former which is usually sought. The decision by a patient as to when a changing stimulus becomes painful is influenced by many other factors, notably by the degree of attention, by apprehension, by previous experience, and also by fatigue. Some drugs also produce an indifference, so that the pain stimulus may be appreciated but fail to elicit a response under these circumstances. Where the patient is already semi-conscious or unconscious, the only threshold which may be determined is that which is required to produce a particular withdrawal response. The stimulus necessary to achieve this, however, is often rather intense and may produce tissue damage.

Because of the strong interaction between the patient and the experimenter, coupled with the possibility of manipulation of the test, it is absolutely vital in this field to use a double-blind method of experimentation, and to include placebos as unknowns to both the patient and the experimenter. All experimental pain methods, with the possible exception of ischaemic pain, take no account of the reaction of the patient to the pain. There is no doubt that it is this component, rather than the absolute threshold, which is principally affected by narcotic analgesics. Reproducibility within ± 10 per cent can be counted as quite good when measuring semi-subjective biological variables.

Measurement of emotional status

A major interest of anaesthetists has been the value of pre-medication. One of the avowed aims of premedication is the relief of anxiety. Not unnaturally, therefore, there has been considerable interest over the years in measuring the degree of anxiety exhibited by patients of various types and ages, and the success of various therapeutic manoeuvres in allaying it. With one or two exceptions, use has been made of the concept that anxiety is associated with changes in the function of the autonomic nervous system, and measurements of the levels of autonomic activity have formed the basis for the measurement of anxiety. Over the years, a large number of possible functions have been evaluated and many of them employed successfully.

It is, of course, perfectly feasible to inquire of the patient as to his state of anxiety and whether it has increased or lessened. It is also possible to observe his demeanour and behaviour and draw similar conclusions. This latter approach has been supplemented by measuring simple parameters of cardiovascular function, most notably the blood pressure and pulse rate. Both of these are elevated when anxiety is present, and a fall following therapy has been interpreted as indicating lessening of anxiety. Nisbet & Norris (1963) evaluated a scoring system incorporating both subjective feelings, observers' opinions, and these simple objective signs. They have discussed the value of each component and the problems associated with the statistical handling of a score derived from such complex and inaccurate variables.

Norris & Telfer (1968) supplemented this technique further by the measurement of forearm blood flow, which they showed to be decreased in states of anxiety. They have also introduced a greater degree of realism into the situation by measuring blood pressure and pulse before and after a stimulus which might be

9

expected to cause mild anxiety, in their case, the application of a face mask. The assumption is implicit that the failure of the pulse and blood pressure to rise after such a stimulus indicates either an adequately sedated patient or one in whom anxiety is not easily aroused.

Other tests based on the activity of the autonomic nervous system have been those involving measurements of skin resistance (Malmo & Shagass 1950) and tissue impedance. A measurement which relies less specifically on autonomic activity and more on the unconscious increased activity in the central nervous system has been the measurement of resting muscle tension (Sainsbury & Gibson 1954).

Since autonomic activity has been widely used as an objective indication of anxiety, it would be naturally advantageous to make a more direct measurement of sympathetic over-activity. Changes in the level of circulating catecholamines would seem a possible approach as yet unexploited, probably because of technical difficulties. Martinez *et al.* (1966) tackled the problem indirectly by measuring the output of catecholamines in the urine. Catecholamine excretion in the urine on the pre-operative day was compared with the catecholamine excretion in a timed period on the day of operation before premedication, and then again with a timed period following premedication. This method is complex and requires a considerably longer period for its application. It is also potentially less sensitive, because short periods of very intense anxiety would not be detected. However, the technique does enable patients who have a continuously high level of anxiety to be detected, and may thus be able to discriminate between the effects of premedication in anxious and non-anxious patients.

It is clearly unprofitable to spend much time attempting to evaluate the effects of anxiety-relieving drugs in patients who are not anxious. Norris & Baird (1967) investigated the incidence of anxiety in a population of 500 patients, and concluded on the basis of questioning and observation of demeanour that 60 per cent showed significant anxiety. Corman *et al.* (1958) using a full psychological questionnaire concluded that over 80 per cent of patients were anxious. However, in the study of catecholamine levels in urine referred to above, less than 15 per cent had abnormally high values. It is clear that what passes for anxiety by psychological standards does not necessarily induce obvious autonomic effects.

Children, with their less sophisticated approach to their feelings, have been a fruitful source for the investigation of drugs for the relief of anxiety. As well as objective views on the child's demeanour, a child by freely weeping or resisting, or by withdrawing his hand from venepuncture, can reveal aspects of anxiety which would be suppressed in an adult. Nevertheless, as before, there is the difficulty of ensuring the validity of the statistical techniques employed in the analysis of the data. Dundee, Moore & Nicholl (1962) in an Appendix, give a worked example of a statistical technique which overcomes some of the disadvantages, and a full discussion is given by Mosteller (1959). The interested reader should not fail to consult the work of Beecher (1959), who has discussed the whole subject of the measurement of subjective responses at length.

REFERENCES

BEECHER H.K. (ed.) (1959) *Measurement of Subjective Responses. Quantitative Effects of Drugs.* Oxford University Press, New York.

CORMAN H.H., HORNICK E.J., KRITCHMAN M. & TERESTMAN N. (1958) Emotional reactions of surgical patients to hospitalization, anesthesia and surgery. *American Journal of Surgery,* **96,** 646.

DUNDEE J.W. & MOORE J. (1960) Alterations in response to somatic pain associated with anaesthesia. I: An evaluation of a method of analgesimetry. *British Journal of Anaesthesia,* **32,** 396.

DUNDEE J.W., MOORE J. & NICHOLL R.M. (1962) Studies of drugs given before anaesthesia. I: A method of pre-operative assessment. *British Journal of Anaesthesia,* **34,** 458.

HEWER A.J.H. & KEELE C.A. (1948) A method of testing analgesics in man. *Lancet,* **2,** 683.

MALMO R.B. & SHAGASS C. (1950) Behavioral and physiologic changes under stress after operations on the frontal lobes. *Archives of Neurology and Psychiatry (Chicago),* **63,** 113.

MARTINEZ L.R., EULER C. VON & NORLANDER O.P. (1966) The sedative effect of premedication as measured by catecholamine excretion. *British Journal of Anaesthesia,* **38,** 780.

MOSTELLER F. (1959) In: *Measurement of Subjective Responses. Quantitative Effects of Drugs* (ed. Beecher H.K.). Oxford University Press, New York.

NISBET H.I.A. & NORRIS W. (1963) Objective measurement of sedation. II: A simple scoring system. *British Journal of Anaesthesia*, **35**, 618.

NORRIS W. & BAIRD W.L.M. (1967) Pre-operative anxiety: A study of the incidence and aetiology. *British Journal of Anaesthesia*, **39**, 503.

NORRIS W. & TELFER A.B.M. (1968) Thalamonal as a pre-operative sedative. *British Journal of Anaesthesia*, **40**, 517.

SAINSBURY P. & GIBSON J.G. (1954) Symptoms of anxiety and tension and the accompanying physiological changes in the muscular system. *Journal of Neurology and Psychiatry*, **17**, 216.

Part III
Handling Numerical Data

16

Descriptive and Deductive Statistics

When it takes a book to provide even an 'Introduction to Statistics', it would be presumptuous to suppose that it is possible to more than skim the subject in two chapters. Nevertheless, the acquisition of numerical data should create an interest in the degree of significance which can be attached to the measurements, and should encourage an appreciation of the techniques of summarising them.

The purpose of this section is to give an outline of the statistical methods which are most used in anaesthesia and in the anaesthetic literature. No initial knowledge of mathematics beyond simple arithemtic and algebra is assumed, and the approach will be to try to explain the scope and purpose of the subject in an intuitive fashion, rather than merely to supply formulae.

The present chapter is concerned with descriptive statistics and with the concepts involved when making deductions about a population from which samples of data have been drawn. The evolution of inferential statistics, such as tests of significance, is discussed in Chapter 17. Throughout both chapters words or phrases which have a special meaning in statistics are written in italics when first used, but they are only defined if the meaning is not clear from the context in which they appear.

Basic terminology

Any observation is termed a *variable*, and in formulae is denoted by x. Any calculation applied to a *sample* of x values, is a *statistic*. Samples are always drawn from a *population*, and any measurement which is representative of a population is a *parameter*.

In statistical terms, a population is a theoretical concept, and is the total number of all similar observations which might have been sampled. In order to derive the characteristics of the population it is necessary to *estimate* the population parameters from the sample statistics. A useful notation convention exists, whereby the theoretical (i.e. original) parameters are denoted by lower-case Greek letters, whereas the estimates of population parameters which are based on samples are given lower-case English letters. Sample statistics, rather confusingly, are often likewise denoted, but in this text, they will be given in full, or in English contractions. For convenience a glossary of the abbreviations used in Chapters 16 and 17 is given in Appendix 1.

DESCRIPTIVE STATISTICS

It is difficult to comprehend the significance of a large body of raw data. If one casts an eye over the values of Po_2 in 100 premedicated individuals, it is possible to get only a rough idea of the average value and scatter of results. Descriptive statistics are designed to express the important features of each group in a way that will enable useful deductions to be made subsequently. They also reduce the bulk of the data, which is of particular practical importance in scientific journals. Descriptive statistics which achieve this reduction are either measures of central tendency or measures of dispersion.

Measures of central tendency

The commonest measure of central tendency is the arithmetic *mean*, or average. The mean is an everyday concept which needs no special explanation. The mean of a group of x values is denoted $\bar{x}$, called x-bar, and is calculated from the equation:

$$\bar{x} = \frac{\sum x}{N}$$

The symbol $\sum$ is the capital 'sigma' and stands for 'the sum of', and 'N' is the number of x values which are added together in order to derive the mean*. The mean tells us around what central value the individual values lie. It also locates the point on a progressive scale around which the values lie. Measures of central tendency are, therefore, sometimes called measures of *location*. If the mean Po_2 of one group is found to be 90 mmHg and the mean of another is found to be 80 mmHg, one is now able to locate where on the scale of Po_2 the two groups lie. The mean values act as representatives of their groups. There are

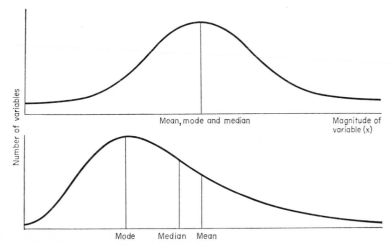

FIG. 16.1. Measures of location. The upper curve is symmetrical and the lower curve is skewed.

other measures of location (Fig. 16.1), such as the *mode* (the most commonly occurring value), the *mid-range* (the middle of the range) and the *median* (the value of the middle observation, when they are arranged in order of size) but they are less commonly used (Fig. 16.1). Still other types of mean may have to be calculated for particular applications but, since they are not

* It is an exceedingly valuable discipline to verbalise any equation on first acquaintance, and see if it appears to 'make sense', and this is particularly necessary when the equation contains many specialised symbols or foreign letters. In this simple instance the equation says, 'to find the average of a group of values, add up all the individual values and divide by the number of values'.

9*

used in deductive statistics, they need not be discussed here.

The mean of a group of values is, perhaps, the easiest statistic to calculate, but this should not encourage its universal employment. If groups of patients are anaesthetised and each group includes infants and octogenarians, the mean ages of the groups, even if different, may have little relevance. Similarly, a mean of 1·8 doses of relaxant per anaesthetic cannot possibly represent any of the actual values which must have all been either one, two, three or more doses. Since the object is description, it is

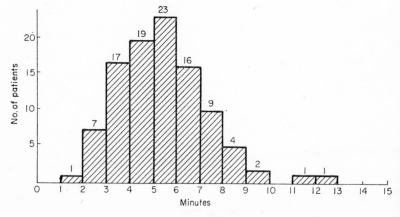

Fig. 16.2. Histogram of sleep time after thiopentone.

more helpful to say how many individuals had each number of doses.

Information of this sort is often best conveyed pictorially as a frequency histogram. Fig. 16.2 is an example. In this case, since all columns are the same width, both the height and area of each column represent the frequency of each occurrence. Such a method of display not only shows clearly which is the commonest value, but also gives a visual impression of the variability of the values. If Fig. 16.2 is compared with Fig. 16.3, for instance, it is clear that not only is the mean sleeping time after propanidid much shorter than with thiopentone, but there is also much less variation between one patient and another.

Measures of dispersion

It would obviously be desirable to have a simple method of expressing the degree of variability of a given set of figures. There are several ways in which variability can be represented, and they all have their uses in different circumstances. For example, it may be appropriate to quote the *range*, that is, the difference

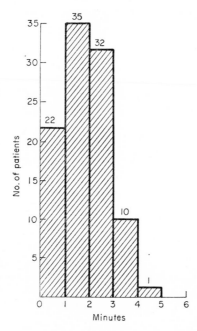

FIG. 16.3. Histogram of sleep time after propanidid.

between the largest and the smallest value. The weakness of this method is that this measurement depends on only two of the values. If one of the subjects in Fig. 16.3 had slept for 10 minutes, the range would have been doubled, but the overall variability of the subjects would have been little different. For this reason one needs some parameter which utilises all the values.

One obvious solution is to subtract each value from the mean value, ignoring the sign, and then to average all these *deviations* from the mean. This value, which is the *mean absolute deviation,** whilst a perfectly valid statistic which uses all the data, has limitations when one wishes to proceed further. For instance, suppose one has a number of values for Po_2 after premedication in two groups of patients; each group will probably have a different mean value, and the variability within each group is also unlikely to be exactly the same. However, we have no reason to suppose that the factors which contribute to that variability, such as sampling technique, electrode response, dial reading errors and biological variation are not the same in each group. Each sample therefore has a variability which can be said *to estimate* the variability in the population from which the sample was drawn. Now, it is frequently desirable to be able to combine both samples to obtain a better estimate of the variability in the population as a whole. However, the mean absolute deviations of the two samples could only be averaged if the means of both samples were the same and there were the same number of observations in each sample. In all other cases to determine the overall mean absolute deviation it would be necessary to calculate the grand mean, and then to recalculate all the deviations of both samples from it.

However, if we *square* all the deviations from the mean before dividing by the number in the sample (N) we obtain the *mean squared deviation*, which is customarily known as the *variance*:

$$\text{var}(x) = \frac{\sum (x - \bar{x})^2}{N}$$

Several practical and theoretical advantages accrue from the use of this concept. Firstly, squaring the differences automatically makes them positive. Secondly, although the terms are derived by squaring the difference between each value and the mean value, the sum of these terms (called the *sum of squares*, or *SS*) can be obtained by a simple method of calculation which does

---

* This is written

$$\frac{\sum |x - \bar{x}|}{N}$$

the parallel lines indicating that the deviation is always taken as positive.

not require a knowledge of the mean value. (The simplified formula is derived in Appendix 2). This has two important consequences.

In the first place, if a measure of variability can be obtained without knowing the mean then it is obviously independent of the mean, and so is a quantity which describes the data in a wholly independent fashion. The importance of this may be illustrated by an example in which two sets of data on the same population are collected by two different observers. If one observer is less careful in collecting the observations than the other, the variability of his data will be greater than that of his more careful colleague. Therefore, the mean squared deviation or variance of the data produced by the careless observer will be greater than the variance of the other set of data. The total variance of a series of observations can thus be apportioned into at least two parts, the underlying variance, and the added observer variance. It can be shown that variances may be added arithmetically and so the variance due to the observer can be deduced by subtracting the underlying variance from the total variance. By an extension of this method, the variance contributed by all the different factors in a group of measurements can be similarly apportioned, this technique being called an *analysis of variance*.

The second practical advantage which accrues from the ability to calculate the variance without knowing the mean, is that it becomes relatively easy to apply tests of significance to data as it accumulates. This is particularly valuable when one is trying to limit the total number of experiments by testing for a significant result after each one. It is merely necessary to add the extra observed value, and the square of the value, to existing columns in the computation and then to divide by the new value of N.

The variance is thus the fundamental, independent measure of variability which can be handled by a simple arithmetical method.

The variance, however, does have the disadvantage that its dimensions are not the same as the original measurements. If the measurements were Po_2 in mmHg, the variance is in $(mmHg)^2$. To obviate this the square-root of the variance is usually taken to give the *standard deviation* (S.D.). The S.D. of a sample, then is defined as:

$$S.D. = \sqrt{\frac{\sum (x - \bar{x})^2}{N}}$$

It can be seen from the formula that, if the majority of the values are near the mean (i.e., $x - \bar{x}$ is small), then the variance and standard deviation are small.

It should be noted that the values for the S.D.'s of different samples do not measure their relative variability. For example, the mean height of a group of men might be 68 inches with an S.D. of 3·1 inches, and that of a group of women might be 59 inches with a S.D. of 2·9 inches. On the face of it, the men appear to be more variable. However, since the means are different, the S.D.'s can only be compared by expressing the S.D. as a percentage of the mean. This quantity is called the *coefficient of variation*. In the case mentioned above the coefficient of variation of men is

$$\frac{3 \cdot 1 \times 100}{68} = 4 \cdot 5 \text{ per cent}$$

and that of women is

$$\frac{2 \cdot 9 \times 100}{59} = 5 \cdot 9 \text{ per cent}$$

so that in fact the height of women, on these figures, is more variable than that of men.

DEDUCTIVE STATISTICS

Although it is convenient to be able to summarise data, the usual reason for making measurements is to discover something about the population from which the sample was drawn. We want to know what is the 'normal' range of fasting blood sugar, or the difference in arterial carbon dioxide tension between patients who have or have not had an epidural injection of local analgesic. These generalizations must be made with varying degrees of confidence, on the basis of the results obtained from the sample. It is for this reason that the design of clinical trials and the selection of subjects is so important. Unless the sample is representative of the population, it is pointless to use sample data to estimate the parameters of the population.

Two kinds of data are commonly subjected to analysis. In one case, the magnitude of each variable could theoretically take any one of an infinite number of values, the number of values being limited only by the accuracy of the measuring instrument. For example, values of Po_2 of 89 mmHg and 91 mmHg, could have been 89·3 mmHg and 90·9 mmHg, or 89·293 mmHg and 90·929 mmHg. Only the limitations of apparatus, time and common sense dictate that one chooses to limit the number of values to, say, whole numbers of millimetres of mercury. Such variables form a *continuous distribution*. On the other hand, the number of radioactive counts recorded on one occasion may be 1007, or 1008, but can never be anything in between. Likewise, either six or seven out of nine patients may complain of pain during an intravenous injection, although such a *discontinuous distribution* may be disguised by reporting it as 66·67 per cent or 77·78 per cent of patients, respectively. In practice, most instrumental measurements yield values which are on a theoretically continuous scale. Even when the distribution of measurements is discontinuous, provided there are a large number of increments and at least thirty or so observations, the statistical methods are essentially similar; consequently, a thorough understanding of the most common continuous distribution, the *'normal'* distribution, is of most value for the beginner.

The normal distribution

If one repeatedly makes some measurement which is subject to random errors, or measures a quantity which is subject to biological variation, and then plots the frequency with which each value occurs, a *frequency distribution curve* is obtained. This has a characteristic 'bell' shape. Figure 16.4, for example, is a hypothetical example showing the frequency with which various values of blood volume are found in 1000 men (a sample large enough to enable us to assume that it is synonymous with the theoretical population). The mean value is 35 ml/kg, the majority of patients falling between 30 and 40 ml/kg. If one wants to know what is the chance of any person taken at random from this population having a blood volume greater than, say, 42

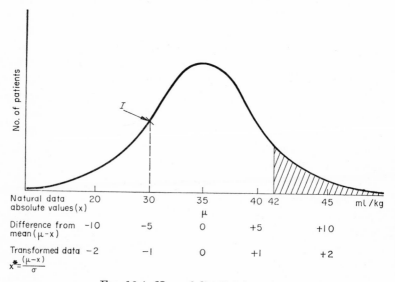

FIG. 16.4. Normal distribution curve.

ml/kg, it can be seen that it corresponds to the proportion of the shaded area under the graph to the whole area.

It would be very laborious to measure or calculate the appropriate area afresh for every such problem. Fortunately, it is not necessary. The equation which describes this curve, although complex, depends on only two variables, the *mean* which locates the curve on the x- (or horizontal) axis, and the *standard deviation* (σ—sigma) which describes its breadth. One standard deviation along the x-axis coincides with the inflection on the curve (marked I in Fig. 16.4) which in this case corresponds to 5 ml/kg, either above or below the mean. The smaller the standard deviation, the taller and narrower the curve is. However, by choosing appropriate scales, all normal curves can be made to look alike; it is merely a matter of expressing each y-value as a percentage and adjusting the x-scale so that the x-value equivalent to one standard deviation is a standard distance away from the mean. The implication of this is that the area under any portion of a normal curve is directly related to the x-values when these are expressed as a *proportion* of the standard deviation.

If we take the mean to be 0, and express the x-values as differences from the mean instead of in absolute quantities, we construct the second x-scale of Fig. 16.4.* If all the differences are then divided by the standard deviation, which is 5 ml/kg in this case, the bottom scale is derived. Tables such as Table 1 in the Statistical Tables (page 306), can now be consulted which give the areas under the curve between various values of our new variable, x^*; x^* is called a *transformed variable* and the formula for its calculation is:

$$x^* = \frac{(x - \mu)}{\sigma}$$

For example, the area between $-2x^*$ and $+2x^*$ is 96 per cent of the total. Five per cent of the area lies outside the range $-1 \cdot 96x^*$ to $+1 \cdot 96x^*$ and so on. Thus by quoting the mean and standard deviation of a population, we are in a position to predict what proportion of individual values will fall within specified limits, or what is the *probability* of obtaining a value falling outside certain limits.

Sampling from a normal population

In the first part of this chapter it was shown that the mean and standard deviation could be used to describe a sample or a population. Usually the population parameters are unknown and one wishes to estimate the population parameters from the

* The Greek 'm', μ (pronounced 'mew'), is used because we are talking about a population.

characteristics of a sample. The question that immediately arises is, 'What *confidence* can we ascribe to such estimates?'. To answer this it is convenient to assume, for the moment, that we have the data from a population and work backwards, asking what we should find if we took samples of varying sizes.

Although Fig. 16.4 represents the data of a population, it could equally well be regarded as a frequency distribution of the *means of samples* of one (N = 1), that is to say that the curve is a plot of the frequency with which each sample mean would occur when each sample consisted of one measurement. (Of course, the mean value ($\bar{x}$) and the value itself (x) are the same thing in a sample of one but it illustrates a method of thinking about the problem). We have already seen that if we know the population parameters, we can assert that 96 out of 100 random sample values will lie within ± 2 S.D. of the mean. Suppose however that the samples each contained ten values taken at random from the population. Simple intuition tells us that the mean value of such a sample ($\bar{x}$) would be more likely to approximate to the population mean (μ) than would any individual value. As in the case of a sample of one, plotting the frequency of means of ten values would also give a normal distribution curve. The mean value of this distribution would inevitably be the same as the population mean from which the samples were drawn, but if plotted on the same scale, the curve of $\bar{x}$ values based on samples of ten would be much narrower than the curve based on samples of one. The narrowing of the distribution curve is the graphical representation of the likelihood that any individual mean value is more likely to approximate to the true underlying mean. That is to say the means of samples of ten would have less variance than the means of samples of one. In Fig. 16.5 such a curve has been superimposed over the original curve of Fig. 16.4. If samples of a hundred were taken, the means would be even closer to the population mean, with even less variability than the means of ten measurements. To get a mental picture of this, try to imagine the problem of estimating the mean height of men of 21 in the population, first by measuring one man, then by measuring ten at a time, and then by taking a hundred at a time. The more measurements in the sample, the nearer to the 'true' mean will the answer be likely to lie, and the tighter will the answers cluster round that value if one repeats the process several times. It is an important theorem of statistics which gives mathematical form to this instinctively perceived generalization, that

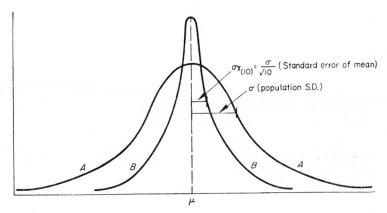

Fig. 16.5. Frequency distribution curve of samples of different sizes.

the *variance of the mean of a sample from a population* is equal to the population variance (σ^2) divided by the number in the sample:

$$\text{var}\,(\bar{x}) = \frac{\sigma^2}{N}$$

Since the standard deviation is the square root of the variance, it follows that the standard deviation of the mean of a sample is equal to the square root of the variance of the mean of a sample or:

$$\text{S.D.}\,(\bar{x}) = \sqrt{\frac{\sigma^2}{N}} = \frac{\sigma}{\sqrt{N}}$$

This statistic, then, is a tool for predicting how nearly the sample mean is likely to approximate to the true (population) mean, and it incorporates both the inherent variability of the individual values in the population and the size of the sample. The variability, and hence the possible error, increases as population variance increases, but decreases as sample size increases. This statistic is usually called the *standard error of the mean (S.E.M.)* or sometimes just the *standard error*. It can equally well be regarded as the standard deviation of the mean of a sample [S.D.($\bar{x}$)].

In order to calculate the range within which the true (population) mean will lie at any desired level of probability one applies similar reasoning to that applied to a population of single values (page 263). We can therefore say that only once in twenty times will this sample mean, or the mean of other comparable samples, be more than 1·96 × the S.E.M. above or below the population mean (μ). This is the same as saying that 95 per cent of all such sample means fall within the range $\mu \pm 1\cdot96 \times$ S.E.M.

It will be noted, however, that in deriving the above formula for the standard error of the mean [S.D.($\bar{x}$)], we have *assumed* that we *know* the population variance (σ^2). Since, on theoretical grounds, we can never know this, it is necessary to *estimate* it as best as we can from the sample data. If the sample is large (more than about 30 observations) then no practical error will arise if one assumes that the sample statistics are the same as the population parameters, and therefore the sample mean and variance of such samples can be used as population mean and variance.

However, when the samples are small this is not acceptable. The sample mean ($\bar{x}$) is still the best estimate that can be obtained of the population mean (μ), but the sample variance almost always *under-estimates* the population variance. The reason for this is that the value of the mean derived from the sample is unlikely to exactly coincide with the true population mean, and therefore the deviations (which are squared, summed and averaged to get the variance) should all have been calculated by taking the values away from the unknown, but slightly different value, for the true mean of the population. It makes no difference whether the population mean is higher or lower than the sample mean, the sum of squared deviations will always be *greater* when the values are subtracted from the true mean of the population rather than from the sample mean.* If one divides the sum of squared deviations by $N - 1$, instead of N, a larger calculated value for the variance is obtained, and it can be shown that this value is more likely to approximate to the true population variance than the original sample variance.

Note that when N is large, say over 30, this correction makes virtually no difference, which is another way of saying that sample statistics for big samples can be freely used as population parameters.

One can accordingly estimate the population variance from any sample size as

$$s^2 = \frac{\sum (x - \bar{x})^2}{N - 1}$$

(s^2 is used instead of σ^2 because this is an *estimate* of the population variance based on a sample.) If it is now assumed that the sample mean is the best estimate of the population mean, then the best estimate for the standard error of the sample mean ($s_{\bar{x}}$) is

$$\text{S.E.M. } (s_{\bar{x}}) = \sqrt{\frac{s^2}{N}} \qquad \text{(cf. page 265)}$$

---

* Suppose the sample values were 2, 2, 3, 4, 8, 5; $N = 6$.

$$\sum (x) = 2 + 2 + 3 + 4 + 8 + 5 = 24, \qquad \bar{x} = 24 \div 6 = 4$$

$$\sum (x - \bar{x})^2 = (4 - 2)^2 + (4 - 2)^2 + (4 - 3)^2 + (4 - 4)^2 + (8 - 4)^2 + (5 - 4)^2$$
$$= 2^2 + 2^2 + 1^2 + 0^2 + 4^2 + 1^2$$
$$= 26$$
$$\therefore \text{ var } (x) = 26 \div 6 = \underline{4 \cdot 3}$$

Suppose now that the true mean of the population from which the above sample of data was drawn, was 5.

The 'true' calculation would have been:

$$\sum (x - \mu)^2 = (5 - 2)^2 + (5 - 2)^2 + (5 - 3)^2 + (5 - 4)^2 + (8 - 5)^2 + (5 - 5)^2$$
$$= 3^2 + 3^2 + 2^2 + 1^2 + 3^2 + 0^2$$
$$= 32$$
$$\sigma^2 = 32 \div 6 = \underline{5 \cdot 3}$$

If the 'true' mean had been 3, the result would still have been 5·3, i.e. the population variance is always greater than the sample variance if the population and sample means do not coincide.

and therefore substituting for s^2

$$\text{S.E.M.} \ (s_{\bar{x}}) = \sqrt{\frac{\sum (x - \bar{x})^2}{(N-1)/N}}$$

The S.E.M. calculated above, then, is a statistic which indicates the degree of reliability with which we can regard the sample mean as representing the true mean. Just as 96 per cent of all values in the sample lie within ± 2 S.D. of the mean, so there is a 96 per cent chance that the population mean will lie within ± 2 S.E.M. of the sample mean. This statistic is used in the calculation of confidence intervals, and in tests of significance, as outlined in the next chapter.

Although we have started from the assumption of a normally distributed population of values, it can be shown that even if the population is *not* normal, the means of samples of a reasonable size (over 30) *are* normally distributed, thus allowing this kind of deduction without postulating a normally distributed population of values.

Methods of reporting quantitative data
It is relevant at this point to consider what statistics should be quoted in scientific papers when the data are too numerous to be given in full. The basic principle is that enough data should be provided to enable the reader to calculate further statistics for himself. This is satisfied by quoting at least the mean, the number of observations and either the standard deviation or the variance. The provision of further information is largely dependent on the conclusions one is trying to draw, and where the major interest resides. If the variability of the data is of interest it is helpful to quote the coefficient of variation; if the interest in the mean is in its use as an indication of the likely true value of the mean of the population, then the standard error of the mean, depending as it does on the number of observations, will give the reader a better impression of the possible range of the true value.

17

Inferential Statistics

It was shown in the previous chapter that the calculation of the mean, variance and standard error of the mean on a sample enables us to infer something concerning the population, and to give a numerical value to the range in which the mean of any sample of similar data will lie at any desired level of probability. The concept of probability is quite an everyday one; in statistical nomenclature it is always denoted by P, and expressed on a scale from 0 to 1. $P = 0$ means that an *event* never occurs, and $P = 1$ implies that it always occurs. $P = 0.5$ describes a situation in which an event is as likely as not to occur. The probability of tossing heads when spinning a coin is 0.5. The sum of all possible outcomes of mutually exclusive events comes to $P = 1$. In some situations such as coin tossing, or card selection, the probability of certain events can be worked out in advance. In medical work this is rarely the case, and by probability one can only mean the frequency of an event to which all *trials* tend to converge in the long term. Examples of this are the five-year survival of a certain disease, or the operative mortality of a particular procedure. In the previous chapter, the probabilities were neither inherently predictable, not dependent on long-term experience, but were mathematical predictions based on a particular sample. In asserting that 95 per cent of all means of samples of a given size will be within 1.96 times the standard error of the mean, one is inevitably implying that the real situation is adequately represented by the mathematical notion of the normal distribution; if a particular sample has a mean outside that range, one can claim that the probability of drawing such a sample at random from a normal population is less than once in twenty times. P is less than 0.05 ($P < 0.05$) and this is therefore asserted to be a *significant* difference which may then be ascribed to special factors, such as treatment, or age. Note, however, that once in every twenty identical experiments such a result *could* occur in the absence of any difference between the sample and the population. A significant result is not certainly true. Once in every twenty times we shall assert a significant effect when in fact none exists, merely on the results of sampling error. This false positive is called a type-α (alpha) error, and this is the value usually chosen when selecting a level of significance. A more stringent level of significance would be a lower P value, i.e., $P < 0.01$, which would assert that there is only one chance in a hundred of making a type-α error, i.e., of falsely concluding that the result was significant when in fact it was due to random sampling effects.

It might be thought that it would be desirable to select a very low value of P, to minimise the possibility of this error. This is not necessarily so, for there is another kind of error over which the experimenter has less control, this is called a type-β (beta) error. This error occurs when it is concluded that there is no difference between the treatment group and the control group, when in fact a difference does exist, i.e. a false negative. The probability of making this error depends on the interaction of two effects. The first is the magnitude of α error that has been selected. The smaller this is, the further out into the 'tail' of the distribution curve a result has to fall before it is considered 'significant'. This leaves a bigger range of potentially real differences which would normally be regarded as being due to the effects of random sampling. If the difference between the populations of treated and non-treated patients is not great, the two distributions overlap to a considerable extent. This difference can then only be resolved by taking larger samples since this causes curves of the sample means to become taller and narrower, so that the overlap of the two distributions is reduced.

Thus we have a two-way conflict. We can increase the likelihood that we do not make an unjustifiable conclusion that treatment is effective by taking a very low level of α, but only at the cost of not detecting real but small effects. We can only avoid this conflict by taking bigger samples, which means more experiments, more expenditure of time, money and patient material. It is customary in biological work to make α, and therefore P to be 0·05, and let β be what it will on the assumption that it is not worthwhile to expend a great effort to unearth minor changes. Conversely, when the experiments are costly or difficult to perform, a higher level of P, say $P = 0·1$, might be quite acceptable, particularly when the consequences of falsely assuming that the treatment is beneficial are not likely to be harmful.

Remember, $P = 0·15$ is conventionally non-significant, and the reader is inclined to dismiss it entirely. However, although there are fifteen chances in a hundred that the result could have occurred by chance, there are eighty-five chances that it did not, and such a value may, on occasion, be enough to justify the acquisition of more data.

Confidence intervals

In the previous chapter it was shown how the values comprising the population of a normal frequency distribution curve could be transformed to special units (x^*), which were derived by taking the difference between each value and the mean, and dividing by the standard deviation:

$$x^* = \frac{|x - \mu|}{\sigma}$$

In this way each value was expressed in terms of how many standard deviations it was away from the mean.

It was also explained that the means of large samples taken from the normal population are themselves normally distributed. It was shown that a curve of such means had a standard deviatio which was equal to the population standard deviation divided by $\sqrt{N}$ and that this statistic is usually called the standard error of the mean (S.E.M.). It is obviously possible to express the sample mean values ($\bar{x}$) comprising such a curve in terms of transformed units also. The values are the means of samples ($\bar{x}$), the mean is the population mean (μ) and the standard deviation of the ($\bar{x}$) values is the standard error. The above formula then becomes:

$$\bar{x}^* = \frac{|\bar{x} - \mu|}{\sigma_{\bar{x}}}$$

Bearing in mind that $\bar{x}$ may be either larger or smaller than μ, this can be arranged algebraically as:

$$\mu = \bar{x} \pm \bar{x}^*(\sigma_{\bar{x}})$$

This equation tells us that the true mean of the population (μ) lies between limits either side of the sample mean ($\bar{x}$), and these limits depend on the chosen value for x^*, and the calculated value of the standard error of the mean ($\sigma_{\bar{x}}$). The value of x^* which is selected depends on the probability, and hence the area, we wish to choose. For an area containing 95 per cent of all values the x^* value is 1·96, and for 99 per cent of all values the x^* value is 2·58. Thus we are able to say that the true mean value of the population (μ) lies between the sample mean ($\bar{x}$) $\pm$ 1·96$\sigma_{\bar{x}}$ with 95 per cent confidence. This implies the alternative that on one occasion in twenty, the true mean will lie outside this range.

The foregoing is correct if the sample size is large and if the population variance can be taken to be the same as the sample variance. However, with small samples, *the means are not distributed normally*, and for each succeedingly smaller sample size the curve becomes slightly flatter and broader. Consequently, one needs to take a bigger value than the x^* value to encompass a given area. These curves have an area distribution which has been tabulated for all sample sizes, and a variable which is analogous to x^* has been computed for each one. This is the 't' distribution.

By analogy with the formula given above

$$t = \frac{|\bar{x} - \mu|}{s_{\bar{x}}}$$

which can likewise be rearranged as follows:

$$\mu = \bar{x} \pm t(s_{\bar{x}})$$

$s_{\bar{x}}$ (the standard error of the mean) is derived, as outlined previously, by estimating the population variance from the sample data, i.e.,

$$s_{\bar{x}} = \sqrt{\frac{\sum (x - \bar{x})^2}{(N - 1)/N}}$$

The value of t chosen for any required area is obtained from a table such as Table 3 in the Statistical Tables, which gives the most commonly used values for each level of significance and for each sample size. Sample size is listed as *degrees of freedom*, a term which will occur again. It refers to the number of items in the data which can vary. Once the mean is specified, $N - 1$ items could vary without changing the mean value, but the last value would be predetermined by the others and the mean. In a collection of numerical data, therefore, the degrees of freedom (DF) are one less than the sample size. The procedure, then, is to find the t-value for the correct degrees of freedom, for the desired area (i.e. probability); this will give the desired *confidence interval for the mean*. For example, with a sample of four values (3 DF) the 95 per cent area is $\pm 3\cdot 18$ ($s_{\bar{x}}$). This should be compared with the normal distribution curve values as given by the formula:

$$\mu = \bar{x} \pm \bar{x}^* . (\sigma_{\bar{x}}) \qquad \text{(see page 272)}$$

when for 95 per cent area x^* was $\pm 1\cdot 96$. The t value is much greater than the x^* value because the distribution curve of the means of samples of only four is much flatter and broader than the normal curve, and therefore a greater distance along the x axis is necessary to encompass the same area.

Note that when DF is 60, the 95 per cent area for $t = 2\cdot 00$, and the t distribution becomes almost synonymous with a normal distribution, as one would expect. ($t = x^*$ at infinity, but for all practical purposes they are identical when there are more than 30 values in the sample.) The formula:

$$\mu = \bar{x} \pm t(s_{\bar{x}})$$

is thus generally applicable irrespective of sample size.

Tests of significance—Student's 't'

One of the commonest situations which presents itself is the possession of data related to two or more fairly small samples, and the question that arises is whether or not they differ significantly from each other. Common sense tells us that the greater the difference between the mean values of the two groups, the less likely they are to be from the same parent population. Similarly, the more values the individual means are derived from, the more reliance we can place on the difference between them. If we divide the actual difference between the means by 'the standard error of this difference' (remember that a 'standard error' is a quantity which decreases as the sample size increases) we can compute a figure which will be larger both when the actual difference is larger and when the sample size is larger. This statistic is Student's 't' and is computed using the formula

$$t = \frac{|\bar{x} - \bar{x}'|}{s_{(\bar{x} - \bar{x}')}}$$

where $|\bar{x} - \bar{x}'|$ is the absolute difference between the sample means, and $s_{(\bar{x} - \bar{x}')}$ is an estimate of the standard error of the difference between the means. The numerator of this fraction is self evident; it is the denominator that requires a moment's analysis.

What hypothesis is being tested? As is so often the case, one puts up the *null hypothesis* that there is really no difference between the samples. If this were so, the mean and the variance of both samples would be similar, although of course one would be surprised if they were identical in small samples. The hypothesis, then, is that the difference between the means is really zero, and the variance of the two samples is the same, i.e., the factors that contribute to the variability are the same in both samples. The first step is to show that the variances are effectively the same.

If the variance of the two samples were identical, the ratio of one to the other would be unity. As the variances increasingly differ, dividing the larger variance by the smaller will give an increasingly large number. There comes a time when the number so obtained is so big that one is forced to conclude that the samples are from different populations, and a straight comparison of their means is not valid. This is the basis of the variance ratio, or F-test. Again sample size must be relevant, since the inherently greater variability of small samples must be allowed for, so the table for the appropriate degree of significance is entered with the degrees of freedom appropriate to each sample, and if the variance ratio is *less* than the value tabulated (Table 2 in the Statistical Tables) then the variances are sufficiently similar to allow one to assume that they are from the same population, and one is at liberty to proceed with the analysis.

The next logical step is to argue that since the two samples have similar variances, combining the data would give a better estimate of the population variance than could be obtained from each individual sample alone. It will be recalled that the best estimate of population variance is obtained by dividing the sum of the squared deviations by $N - 1$. In this case we can add the sum of squared deviations (SS) for each sample, and divide by $N - 1$ for each sample.

$$s^2 = \frac{SS + SS'}{(N - 1) + (N' - 1)}$$

Having calculated the best estimate of the population variance we can use it to obtain a more accurate value for the variance ($s_{\bar{x}}^2$) and standard error ($s_{\bar{x}}$) of each sample mean by dividing by the number in that sample:

$$s_{\bar{x}}^2 = \frac{s^2}{N} \qquad \text{S.E.M. } (s_{\bar{x}}) = \frac{s}{\sqrt{N}}$$

and

$$s_{\bar{x}'}^2 = \frac{s^2}{N'} \qquad \text{S.E.M. } (s_{\bar{x}'}) = \frac{s}{\sqrt{N'}}$$

We now have the standard errors of the means of each sample; what is the standard error of the difference between the means? Again, it is best to look at the problem intuitively. If both the standard errors are very small, the true mean of each sample lies between small limits. The difference between the two mean values is therefore known fairly accurately, and the standard error of the difference (which delineates the range within which the true difference lies) will also be small. For example, if there is a 95 per cent probability that the mean weight of one group of men lies between 69·8 kg and 70·2 kg, and the mean weight of another group lies between 70·2 kg and 70·6 kg, then we feel 95 per cent confident that the true difference lies between the smallest and largest probable differences, i.e. 0 and 0·8 kg. If, however, the standard error of one group is large, the possible range for the difference increases. When both groups have large standard errors, the possible range for the true mean of the difference between the two means becomes doubly large.

Unfortunately, we cannot just add the two standard errors, but as was emphasised earlier, variances *can* be combined arithmetically, and if we add the two variances we get what could be called the variance of the difference, e.g.,

$$s_{(\bar{x}-\bar{x}')}{}^2 = \frac{s^2}{N} + \frac{s^2}{N'}$$

If the samples are the same size, this simplifies to:

$$s_{(\bar{x}-\bar{x}')}{}^2 = \frac{2s^2}{N}$$

The standard error of the difference is therefore the square root of this quantity. This is the denominator of our fraction

$$t = \frac{|\bar{x} - \bar{x}'|}{s_{(\bar{x}-\bar{x}')}}$$

i.e.

$$t = \frac{|\bar{x} - \bar{x}'|}{\sqrt{\dfrac{s^2}{N} + \dfrac{s^2}{N'}}}$$

It has already been suggested that both a *large* difference in means and a *small* standard error of the difference increase the likelihood that the difference is significant, and this formula

shows that both of these conditions will lead to larger values of
t. If, therefore, the table of t-values (Table 3 in the Statistical
Tables) is entered for the desired area (or P value) using the
degrees of freedom contributed by both samples $[(N - 1)$
$+ (N' - 1)]$ and if the value in the tables is *exceeded* by the
calculated value, then the difference is significant at that P value,
and the null hypothesis is rejected. A worked example may be
found in Appendix 3.

t-test for paired observations
The foregoing is often called an unpaired t-test because we are
working on data derived from dissimilar samples which may have
been drawn from different populations. In some experimental
situations it is possible to have data on two successive occasions
in the same individual. For example, one may wish to compare
the pulse rate before and after atropine. In this situation the
'between patient' variability is eliminated and one would expect
to be able to detect much smaller differences. Instead of working
with differences between the mean values of the two groups, one
can work with the actual differences themselves. The null hypothesis is that there is a population of differences, with a mean
difference of zero, and that the sample of differences which we
have found could have occurred at random. The principle of the
calculation follows the same logic as before. There is, in fact, a
mean of the differences between the two sets of values ($\bar{d}$) whose
value is not zero; if we divide this mean difference by the
standard error of the difference ($s_{\bar{d}}$), we shall again get a t-value.
The more the difference departs from zero the more likely is it
to be significant, and the higher the t-value. Similarly, the more
consistent the differences, and the more numerous the observations, the smaller will be the standard error of the difference and
the higher the t-value. For paired samples, therefore,

$$t = \frac{\bar{d}}{s_{\bar{d}}}$$

Again the numerator, the mean difference, presents no problem; the denominator is simply the square root of the best

estimate of the variance of the population of differences, divided by the number of observations (cf. page 268).

$$s_{\bar{d}} = \sqrt{\frac{\sum (d - \bar{d})^2}{(N - 1)/N}}$$

The table of t values is entered with the appropriate DF which in this case is one less than the total number of *differences* (not two less than the total number of observations) and at the appropriate value of P. A worked example may be found in Appendix 3.

One and two-tailed tests

In the preceding sections the problem was to determine whether or not the means of the two samples were significantly different, and this was done by comparing the magnitude of the difference with an estimate of the variability of the difference. No consideration was given to the problem of which of the two means was the larger for one was only interested in establishing that, at a chosen level of probability, the difference was outside the limits that could have occurred by chance in samples of that size and variability. The appropriate area under the t-distribution curve was therefore equally divided between both 'tails' of the distribution, and in the case of $P = 0.05$, there would have been a probability of $P = 0.025$, that A was larger than B, and $P = 0.025$ that B was larger than A. This is therefore called a 'two-tailed' test of significance.

Quite commonly, however, one has good reasons for expecting one mean to be greater than another. Indeed, it may only make clinical sense for one mean to be greater than the other. In this situation one should apply a one-tailed test and show that the value is in the appropriate area at one end of the curve. The t-value that is associated with 5 per cent of the area at one end is, of course, the value that is tabulated for twice that area when distributed over both ends of the curve, or $P = 0.10$. This is always a *smaller* value of t, i.e. one easier to exceed.

Non-parametric tests for continuously variable data

So far the discussion has centred around tests of significance which have been dependent on the actual values of variables which could theoretically take any value on a continuous spectrum. Much simpler and quicker tests of significance can be applied which do not depend on the actual values themselves. These inevitably are less powerful tools and may fail to reveal significant differences which a *t*-test would detect. However, their ease makes them useful for an initial analysis, and if they yield significant results, the more laborious *t*-test would certainly do so too. An example of a *non-parametric* test is the Willcoxon two-sample rank test. In comparing two groups of data, $x_1, x_2, ..., x_N, x'_1, x'_2, ..., x'_N$ all the values from both groups are arranged in order of increasing magnitude. Then for every x value, the total number of x' values which precede it are counted, and all the resulting totals are added together. For example, if one group of Po_2 values (x) in millimetres of mercury were 91, 88, 67, 96, 83, and the other group (x') were 82, 77, 69, 90, 66, they are arranged 66, 67, 69, 77, 82, 83, 88, 90, 91, 96 (x values underlined). The first x value is preceded by one x' value. The second and third x values are preceded by four x' values and the fourth and fifth x values, are preceded by five x' values. The total of x' values which precede the x values is therefore $1 + 4 + 4 + 5 + 5 = 19$. Now if both samples had been drawn at random from a single population, there would be just as many x values preceding x' values, as x' values preceding x values, and both ways of computing would give a similar total. (The two totals, incidentally, will add up to $N \times N'$, and so only one computation need be done.) If on the other hand, the two samples were from widely separated populations, all of one group of values might precede the first of the other group, and one total would equal $N \times N'$, and the other would be zero. This would obviously be a significant result, whereas roughly equal values would indicate that there was probably no real difference. The significance of an intermediate result can be determined by reference to the appropriate tables.

10

Previous discussion has centred around the analysis of continuous variables, which are theoretically able to assume any value.

Some types of data, however, are discontinuous. For example, radioactive counts can never be other than whole numbers, and the proportion of patients who develop a sore throat following intubation will be based on a whole-number sample. There are two mathematical distributions which can be used as models to represent most examples of discontinuous data. These are the binomial and Poisson distributions.

The binomial distribution
This is a special, simple case of a more general distribution, the multinomial distribution. It is applicable to all 'either/or' situations. If a population contains items or subjects which belong to one of two mutually exclusive categories, it is a binomial population. The categories may be cured/not cured; awake/ asleep; dead/alive; male/female, or any pair in which, if a variable is in one group, it is not in the other. If one wishes to describe the characteristics of such a population, there is only one parameter, namely the proportion of each component. It will be recalled that in a population of quantitative data, the composition of *samples* was described by quoting both the mean and the variance, and these quantities could vary quite independently. In a sample drawn from a binomial population this is not so, and both depend only on the proportions of each in the population. To try and get a mental picture of this, imagine a population, say, of 10,000 billiard balls, of which only 2 per cent are white, the rest black. In any random selection of one ball, there would be 98 chances of drawing black to 2 chances of drawing white. Suppose one were to draw samples of, say, 100 balls at random. We should expect to get 98 black and 2 white, but would on occasions get 99 or 97 black with 1 or 3 white. It would be distinctly rare to get 96 or 100 black, and 95 black with 5 white would be most unusual. Note that it is impossible to get more than 100 black, but possible to get less than 96. The distribution

is therefore markedly *skewed* (see Fig. 16.1), and also extremely narrow; its variance is obviously small.

Suppose now, that the population is 50:50 white and black. In samples of 100 at random, one would expect to get 50:50 more often than any other proportion, but 45:55, or even 40:60 would not occasion great surprise. In this instance the distribution is not skewed, and intuitively one can see that if the samples are reasonably large, the proportions found in the samples would look remarkably like a normal distribution. Furthermore, the variance is much larger than in the case of the 98:2 population. It can be shown that the variance of a binomial population is equal to the product of the proportions of the two constituents of the population. The variance of a sample, as usual, depends both on the variance of the population from which it is drawn, and the size of the sample.

$$\text{sample variance} = \frac{\sigma^2}{N}$$

In the case of a sample of 100 taken from a population of billiard balls in which 2 per cent are white, this equals

$$\frac{98 \times 2}{100} = 1 \cdot 96$$

Therefore, the standard deviation S.D. $= \sqrt{1 \cdot 96} = 1 \cdot 4$. With a sample of 100 taken from a 50:50 population the variance would be

$$\frac{50 \times 50}{100} = 25$$

and the S.D. is therefore $\sqrt{25} = 5$.

Thus if the proportions of the two components are very different, the sampling distribution is skewed and the variance is small, but as the proportions become more equal, the sampling distribution resembles the normal curve and the variance becomes larger.

A further characteristic of samples from a binomial distribution is that the sampling distribution not only depends on the population parameters, but also depends on the size of the sample. Again, to get a mental picture of this, suppose the proportions were 9:1 black to white; then a sample of 10 could be 9:1 (most common), 10:0, and 8:2 (less common), 7:3 or less white (increasingly rare, in fact, an obviously skewed distribution). If one increases the sample size to 100, but keeps the underlying population parameters the same, what happens? The most common sample would be 90:10, less common 89:11 or 91:9, less common again 88:12 and 92:8 and so on, but in a big sample like this it would be extremely uncommon to be outside the limits: 84–96 black.* Note that this has resulted in a virtually normal, unskewed distribution *merely as a result of increasing the sample size.*

As the relative proportions in the population differ more widely, it needs a larger sample to make the sampling distribution reasonably normal. As an approximation, the expected number of either category in a sample must be at least five if a reasonably normal distribution is to occur. So if only 10 per cent of the population falls into one category, then the sample must contain at least 50 items (50 × 10 ÷ 100 = 5). One can see that the normal distribution, although belonging to continuously variable data, is versatile enough to be applicable to many binomial populations.

Small binomial samples—sequential analysis
When the expected number in one category is less than five, other methods of calculating the expected composition of samples must be employed. The kind of situation in which this might arise is where a new treatment with a potentially serious complication such as aplastic anaemia is to be tried out in a disease with a high natural mortality. It is obviously essential to show an improvement with the smallest number of experiments, and therefore, potentially with less than five patients in one of the categories. This sort of problem is not commonly encountered in

* Roughly

$$s = \sqrt{\frac{90 \times 10}{100}} = 3$$

95 per cent confidence limits = 90 ± (2 × 3) = 90 ± 6.

the anaesthetic literature, and the methods appropriate to its solution will not be discussed here. The reader should consult one of the books listed in the Bibliography.

There is, however, a simple application related to the binomial distribution which has recently come into vogue, and this is the use of sequential analysis charts. These charts can be used only in an either/or situation. They are of most value in comparing two drugs, or procedures, with regard to a single outcome. The assessment is based simply on a decision that the outcome of treatment A is better, or worse, than the outcome of treatment

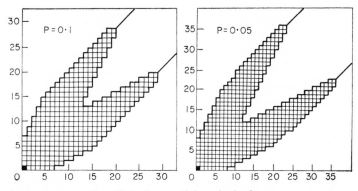

Fig. 17.1. Sequential analysis chart.

B, or that no difference can be detected. Matched pairs of patients are entered into the trial, and one receives treatment A and the other treatment B, according to a random selection process, such as tossing a coin. The chart is entered at the bottom left-hand corner, and after the first pair have received their respective treatments, a cross is drawn on the square vertically above the black square if treatment A is superior, and horizontally to the right if treatment B is superior (see Fig. 17.1). If there is no difference, no entry is made. A second pair is then entered into the trial and the process repeated. When the line of crosses so constructed passes over either of the lateral limits, that treatment is statistically superior to the other. The numbers

of squares within the bounds are specific for the level of significance which is desired, and $P = 0.05$ and $P = 0.1$ charts are
both available. If the middle boundary is crossed, no significant
difference can be detected. A full analysis of the method can be
consulted in Armitage (1960).

Chi-squared test*

There are some situations in which it is possible to compare the
observed results of an experiment with what might have been
expected. Expectation in this context may take various forms.
If a new treatment is being tried in a condition in which the
complication rate is known and fairly constant, the expectation
on the null hypothesis is that the complication rate will be
unaltered by the treatment. A statistical test which can be
applied in a large number of such situations is the chi-squared
test. This has the further advantage that it can be applied to
more than two categories of outcome, and it is thus possible to
evaluate the significance of the results in a trial when these
are excellent, good, fair, poor, etc. The simplest case is a comparison between two treatments, each of which is capable of only
two outcomes. For example, suppose a clinical trial was constructed to evaluate the use of meprobamate to prevent suxamethonium pains, and fifty patients were given the active drug,
and fifty a placebo. If the number of patients who developed
pain was recorded, Table 17.1 could be constructed. This is
called a 2×2 contingency table. Each of the entries is the
observed frequency (O). On the null hypothesis, our expectation
is that since forty patients in all developed pain, one could
expect twenty patients in each group to develop pain and thirty
to have no pain. These are the expected frequencies (E). For each
entry in the table the difference between observed and expected
frequencies is squared, and divided by the expected frequency.
χ^2 is the sum of all such terms. Obviously, if the differences are
small, $(E - O)^2/E$ will be small, and this is independent of
sample size. Tables can by consulted for critical values of χ^2

* Chi-squared is pronounced to rhyme with eye, preceded by a hard 'k'
and written χ^2.

TABLE 17.1. A 2×2 contingency table.

	Pain	No pain	Totals
Meprobamate	10 ($E = 20$)	40 ($E = 30$)	50
Placebo	30 ($E = 20$)	20 ($E = 30$)	50
Totals	40	60	100

The observed number (O) is the figure entered in each square of the table. E is the expected number, on the assumption that as 40 patients had pain, there would be 20 in each group if the treatment had no effect.

$$\chi^2 = \sum \frac{[E - O]^2}{E}$$

$$= \frac{[(20 - 10) - 0\cdot5^*]^2}{20} + \frac{[(40 - 30) - 0\cdot5^*]^2}{30}$$

$$+ \frac{[(30 - 20) - 0\cdot5^*]^2}{20} + \frac{[(30 - 20) - 0\cdot5^*]^2}{30}$$

$$= \frac{9\cdot5^2}{20} + \frac{9\cdot5^2}{30} + \frac{9\cdot5^2}{20} + \frac{9\cdot5^2}{30}$$

$$= \frac{2 \times 9\cdot5^2}{20} + \frac{2 \times 9\cdot5^2}{30} = \frac{6 \times 9\cdot5^2}{60} + \frac{4 \times 9\cdot5^2}{60} = \frac{10 \times 9\cdot5^2}{60}$$

$$= \frac{9\cdot5^2}{6} = \frac{90\cdot25}{6} = \underline{15\cdot04}$$

Since this exceeds the tabulated value $10\cdot8$ ($P = 0\cdot001$ for 1 DF), the result is highly significant ($p < 0\cdot001$). See Statistical Table 4.

* Yates' Correction—see Appendix 4.

which are exceeded by chance at various levels of probability (see Table 4 in Statistical Tables). However, the number of categories affects the situation, and the tables are constructed in terms of degrees of freedom. For χ^2 the DF is not one less than the sample size, as in quantitative data, but one less than the number of categories, irrespective of the number of items in each category. Although the results have been laid out as a 2×2 table in the example, there are only two categories (pain/no pain) and so there is only one degree of freedom. This can be confirmed by observing that once one entry is changed, the marginal totals fix all the other entries. Where there are only two categories, as in this example, a simple correction has also to be applied (the Yates correction—see Appendix 4). There is only one restriction, which is similar to that placed on using the normal distribution for a binomial population, namely that the expected number of items in each category must be at least 5. This distribution is most useful when there are more than two outcomes, or when, for example, one is comparing more than two treatments. In such cases a table is constructed in which each square or *cell* refers to one outcome, e.g. 'Treatment B no improvement'. $[(E - O)^2 \div E]$ is calculated for each cell and totalled to give χ^2. Such a table is a 2×3, or 3×3, contingency table, depending on its composition.

The Poisson distribution

The data which have been handled in the previous section have been of the type that either an event occurred, or some alternative event occurred, or at least a recognizable 'non-event' occurred, i.e., the patient did *not* die. There are, however, situations in which events occur in which there is no meaningful measure of the non-events. We can say how many goals are scored in a football match, but there is no way of counting the goals that did not get scored. In medical work, the most common example of this type of data is in the analysis of radioactive counts. One can count the number of disintegrations per minute, but no meaning can be given to the number of 'non-disintegrations'. If one makes replicate counts, there will be a tendency for the results to converge to a mean value, and there will be a variance of the individual counts about this mean. One can see that the greater the number of counts, on any occasion, the more likely is the answer to approach the average count; it is not surprising, therefore, that the variance and hence the standard deviation are a function of the number of counts. It can be shown that the variance is equal to the mean and so the standard deviation depends on the square root of the mean. Consequently the standard deviation becomes a progressively smaller proportion of the total counts as the number of counts increases. Provided that more than 100 counts are recorded, the confidence interval for the mean count can be estimated from a random sample count on lines familiar from the study of a normal curve, namely that the average count lies between the limits:

$$\text{sample count} \pm 1 \cdot 96 \times \sqrt{\text{sample count}}$$

for a 95 per cent confidence interval and,

$$\text{sample count} \pm 2 \cdot 58 \times \sqrt{\text{sample count}}$$

for a 99 per cent confidence interval. The reasoning behind this is gone into in greater detail in Chapter 7.

CORRELATION

Many biological variables are interrelated. The height of children increases with age, the arterial Po_2 decreases with age, the blood volume increases with both height and weight. When the value of one variable can be predicted with greater accuracy when the value of another variable is known, the two variables are said to be *correlated*. If both tend to increase together, they are *positively* correlated and when one decreases as the other increases, they are *negatively* correlated.

There are two traps for the unwary that are particularly applicable to correlation data. The first is that a correlation is merely a mathematical relationship, and there is no certainty that a change in either variable is the cause of a change in the other. Many bizarre but mathematically quite sound correlations

11

exist in which the two variables are both dependent on another factor, or the relationship may be entirely accidental. For example, it is highly likely that a significant positive correlation could be established between the national average number of hours spent watching television, and the mean length of women's skirts.* Such correlations over time are extremely common, and usually fortuitous. In the case quoted, no one would be likely to proceed to argue that the light emitted by television sets has a deleterious effect on the free edges of certain fabrics, but when a biologically plausible 'explanation' exists, an unwarranted cause and effect relationship may be unjustifiably assumed. The second trap is unjustified extrapolation. There is never any reason to assume that the relationship between two variables exists outside the range of data that have been collected. For example, the fact that the height of children increases in a reasonably linear fashion over time, does not enable one to predict the height of 70-year-old people. Again, although common sense would prevent one from making such an obvious error, similar reasoning might lead one to the conclusion that a systolic blood pressure of 80 mmHg would be associated with a lower mortality rate than that found in normal fit individuals.

Displaying correlation data

One common way in which the correlation between variables is displayed is by means of a scatter diagram. Usually an experimenter has a variable which he chooses independently, for example, age or a time interval, which is therefore termed the *independent variable*. The other, the *dependent variable*, is then measured at various values of the independent variable. The independent variable is usually plotted on the x axis and the dependent variable on the y axis. For example, the Po_2 of pre-operative patients has been found to decline with age. In this case, although people of specific ages may not have been sought, it is logical to think of the age as the independent variable and examine how the Po_2 varies with age. It is quite permissible to plot the variation of age with Po_2, but it seems an illogical

* This example may need to be changed in the next edition!

way of visualising the problem. When such results are plotted, there is often a quite obvious trend, and lines can be drawn by eye which appear to fit the points best. This is a slip-shod and possibly misleading procedure, and it is preferable to calculate the best line by methods which will be discussed shortly and then to draw it in.

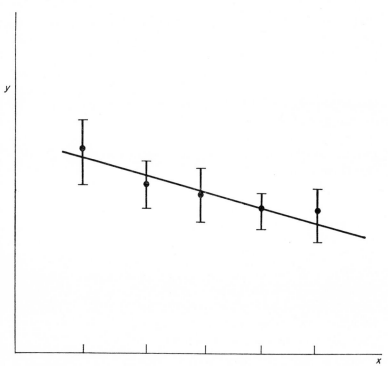

Fig. 17.2. Regression line with standard errors of y values at each x value.

It is quite common for there to be several y values for each x value. It is thus possible to calculate the standard error of the mean of the y values at each x value, and this can be displayed as a vertical line of appropriate length for each value of x, on either side of the mean value (Fig. 17.2). It is easy to be misled by this also. There is a natural tendency to think that the line of best fit will pass through each such line. In fact we know that one S.E.M. will include only about 69 per cent of all large sample means. If the samples are small, the confidence interval will be even greater. For example, if each point on a correlation graph is a mean of four samples, the length of line for 95 per cent confidence should be more than three times one S.E.M. ($t = 3 \cdot 18$ for 3 DF).

It might be supposed that it would be correct, therefore, to plot the mean value, and a vertical line corresponding to a 95 per cent confidence interval for that sample. Certainly the line illustrating the correlation of the two variables (often called the *regression line*) will pass through nineteen out of twenty such lines, but in fact the confidence interval for the line as a whole, depending on the accumulation of all the data, is narrower than the band formed by joining the ends of the lines representing the individual confidence intervals, each of which depends only on a small sample.

Calculation of regression lines

It is necessary to start from the basic assumption that the correlation between the variables x and y (if it exists) is a *linear* one. If we suspect that it is not, it is usually more convenient to plot one variable on a different type of scale, so as to transform the relationship into a linear one rather than to attempt to work on a mathematically more complex relationship. This is of relevance in plotting drug dose/response curves where there is generally a linear response of some tissue to a logarithmic change in concentration of drug.

Figure 17.3 is a simple straight line graph showing a linear correlation. An equation that describes such a line is of the type:

$$y = bx + a$$

where a is the value of y when x is zero, and b is the slope. This tells us that each y-value is b times the appropriate x-value plus or minus a consistent increment. The value of b the slope, is also known as the *regression coefficient*. In any group of experimentally derived values, there will be a scatter of y values above and below the line. It will be recalled that in a footnote to the discussion on the estimation of population variance (page 267), we saw that the mean could be regarded as the value which yielded a minimal value for the sum of squared deviations of the observations from it. By the same reasoning, the mean value, or best estimate of the line is the line for which

$$\sum (y - \tilde{y})^2$$

is a minimum for all the y values. ($\tilde{y}$ is the value of y at the corresponding x value, calculated from the regression equation.) This is the 'least squares line'. To show how the values of a and b

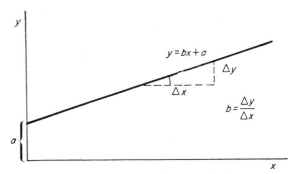

Fig. 17.3. Equation of a straight line.

in a linear equation are calculated to make this quantity a minimum requires a knowledge of elementary differential calculus; however, the principle can be appreciated without it.

First of all, one can accept as reasonable that the line will pass through the value which represents the mean of y and the mean of x, i.e., the general mean. It if did not pass through this point, then clearly the sum of all the squared deviations would be larger. If this is accepted, the value of a in the regression line is immaterial since we now have a fixed point, and once the slope is calculated this will fix the whole line. The slope is obviously some expression which relates an increase or decrease in y values to an increase in x values (Fig. 17.3). It can be thought of as the mean deviation of y divided by the mean deviation of x. It is actually calculated by the formula

$$b \text{ (slope)} = \frac{\sum (x - \bar{x}) . (y - \bar{y})}{\sum (x - \bar{x})^2}$$

The denominator is the sum of squared deviations which is the basis of the calculation of the variance of single parameter variables, and which we have met earlier. The numerator is the sum of the product of the x and y deviations. Like the variance, it can actually be calculated more easily by an alternative formula (see Appendix 5).

Confidence interval of a slope

If the y values varied without any relation to the x values, there would be no correlation and the true slope would be zero. Any random sample of data, however, might yield either a positive or negative slope. If the confidence interval for the slope includes zero slope, then clearly the slope cannot be differentiated from a horizontal line and no true correlation exists. However, before one can calculate the confidence interval for a slope, it is necessary to introduce a new concept.

It will be recalled that it is possible to add variances: in fact the variances of two means were added in order to derive the variance of the difference between them (page 276). From this it is a simple step to the concept that the total variance of data can equally be thought of as the resultant of adding variances which are attributable to various causes. In the case of regression data, consider first what would be the position if all the y values fell exactly on the slope. Under these circumstances, the variance would be the sum of squared deviations of each y value from the mean y value, and the variance of the y values would be entirely that due to regression. However, in any experimental situation, some y values fall on either side of the line, and the sum of squared deviations of the y values from the mean value of y will be greater than it would be if they all fell on the line. The actual variance, therefore, can be regarded as composed of two parts, the variance which arises from regression, and added to it, the variance which results from the scatter of y values above and

below the regression line. This additional variance is known as
the *error variance*. (The square root of the error variance can be
thought of as the standard deviation of individual y values above
and below the regression line.) The error variance, therefore, is
the variance that remains after the variance due to regression
has been subtracted. The error variance is usually designated as

$$s_{y.x}{}^2$$

and the standard deviation of the y values around the regression
line, therefore, is

$$s_{y.x}$$

This quantity can be calculated from formulae which can be
obtained from standard textbooks (one form is included in
Appendix 6).

Having obtained the error variance, one is in a position to
calculate the confidence interval of the slope. The logic in this
is exactly analogous to the logic in determining the confidence
interval for the true mean from a sample of single parameter
data discussed earlier. It is an equation of the type:

$$\mu = \bar{x} \pm t(s_{\bar{x}}) \qquad \text{(see page 272)}$$

in which we calculated the range in which the true mean (μ) lay,
by reference to the sample mean ($\bar{x}$), the S.E .of the mean ($s_{\bar{x}}$), and
the t value appropriate to the degrees of freedom. In the present
case the formula is

$$\beta = b + t \cdot \frac{(s_{y.x})}{\sqrt{SS_x}}$$

β is the true slope, b the slope calculated from the sample data,
$s_{y.x}$ is the square-root of the error variance, and $\sqrt{SS_x}$ the square
root of the sum of squared deviations of the x values.

One can push the analogy between single parameter and
correlation data even further. In the same way that it was
possible to test for the significance between two sample means
with a Student's t test, so one can test whether or not two slopes
differ significantly. In this case, t is equal to the difference
between two *slope* estimates, divided by a term which represents
the standard error of the difference of the slopes. The standard
error is computed by first estimating the population error

variance by pooling the data, and the difference of slope is considered to be significant if a t value is exceeded (the formula is included in Appendix 8).

Correlation coefficient

In any sample of data, the actual angle the slope makes with the x-y axes depends on the scale of the axes upon which the data are plotted. It is not immediately obvious, therefore, whether or not the correlation is strong or weak. What one would like is a measure of correlation that is independent of the actual units of measurement on the x and y scales. We referred earlier to the concept that the total variance of the data was made up of the variance due to regression and the error variance. It is clear that the strength of the correlation is that part of the total variance which is *not* due to the error variance but *is* due to regression. If one divides the regression sum of squares by the total sum of squares one gets a number which may be thought of as a ratio of two variance components. Obviously, if there were no error variance then the regression sum of squares and the total sum of squares would be the same, and this fraction would be 1 or −1, depending on the direction of slope. Similarly, if there were no slope, all the regression would be error sum of squares and the fraction would reduce to zero. It is customary, however, to use the square root of this value, known as the *correlation coefficient* (r), and likewise the value of r may vary from zero, implying no correlation, to −1 or +1. A formula for calculating r is given in Appendix 9. It is now possible to complete the analogy with single parameter data; r is the slope of the regression line when the coordinates of x and y have been transformed, each x value being divided by the standard deviation of x values and the y values divided by the standard deviation of y values. In other words, the scales of both axes have been adjusted in terms of the standard deviation of the measurements, just as any particular set of normally distributed single parameter data could be standardised to produce a standard normal curve in which the x values were plotted in terms of their standard deviation. All slopes with the same correlation coefficient therefore have the same strength of correlation, regardless of the apparent differences between the slopes when based on the original data, just as all similar single parameter data had the same relative coefficient of variation when the actual standard deviation was divided by the mean.

There is no doubt that the formulae and concepts involved in correlation data are by no means so easy to visualise intuitively. Nevertheless, they do arise as logical extensions of concepts which are simpler to grasp with single parameter data. They are yet another area in which an understanding of the construction and implications of the normal distribution curve are vital. This curve is of use even when matters become more complex and correlations between logarithmic and linear variables are attempted.

Statistics should be regarded as a tool. No one can maintain proficiency with a tool merely by observing how it is used and how it is made. Only by using statistics as a tool, can one become familiar with them. As with most kinds of learning, the memory resides in the motor cortex. Even if the reader has been able to follow both these chapters right to their conclusion, it is unlikely he will retain the knowledge for an appreciable time unless he uses it in a practical way. It is to be hoped that the day is not far distant when a calculating machine will be as familiar in an anaesthetic department as a pH meter.

REFERENCE

Armitage P. (1960) *Sequential Medical Trials*. Blackwell Scientific Publications, Oxford and Edinburgh.

FURTHER READING

Bulmer M.G. (1967) *Principles of Statistics*. 2nd ed. Oliver and Boyd, Edinburgh and London.

Dunn O.J. (1967) *Basic Statistics: A Primer for the Biomedical Sciences*. John Wiley & Sons, London.

Goldstein A. (1964). *Biostatistics—An Introductory Text*. The Macmillan Company, New York.

Hill A.B. (1966) *Principles of Medical Statistics*. 8th ed. The Lancet Ltd., London.

Moroney M.J. *Facts from Figures*. Penguin Books Ltd., Harmondsworth, Middlesex.

11*

Appendices

x	Any variable
$\bar{x}$	The arithmetic mean of the x values
N	The number of observations in a sample
var (x)	The variance of a sample
S.D.	Standard deviation of a sample
SS	Sum of squared deviations from the mean
$\sum$	Add up
μ	Population mean ⎫
σ^2	Population variance ⎬ Theoretical
σ	Population standard deviation ⎭
x^*	Value of variable in units of deviation $(x^* = x - \bar{x}/\text{S.D.})$
S.E.M. $(s_{\bar{x}})$	Standard error of the mean
s^2	Estimate of population variance based on sample statistics
s	Estimate of population standard deviation based on sample statistics
DF	Degrees of freedom—the number items of the data which are free to vary
$s_{(\bar{x}-\bar{x}')}$	Standard error of difference between the means of two independent samples
d	A difference between two sequential observations in same patient
$\bar{d}$	Mean of the population of differences
$s_{\bar{d}}$	Standard error of differences
$\tilde{y}$	The value for y calculated from the regression equation

r	The correlation coefficient
$s_{y \cdot x}^{2}$	The error-variance of x and y

APPENDIX 2. A SHORT CUT METHOD FOR COMPUTING THE VARIANCE AND STANDARD DEVIATION

$$\text{variance} = \frac{\sum (x - \bar{x})^2}{N} \tag{1}$$

by definition. The term $\sum (x - \bar{x})^2$ is called the sum of squares (SS) and can be represented as:

$$SS = (x_1 - \bar{x})^2 + (x_2 - \bar{x})^2 + \cdots (x_N - \bar{x})^2 \tag{2}$$

Expanding each term gives:

$$SS = (x_1^2 - 2\bar{x}x_1 + \bar{x}^2) + (x_2^2 - 2\bar{x}x_2 + \bar{x}^2) \cdots (x_N^2 - 2\bar{x}x_N + \bar{x}^2) \tag{3}$$

This may be shortened to:

$$SS = \sum (x^2) - 2\bar{x} \sum (x) + N\bar{x}^2 \tag{4}$$

Now

$$\bar{x} = \frac{\sum (x)}{N}$$

Substituting for $\bar{x}$ in (4) gives:

$$SS = \sum (x^2) - 2\frac{\sum (x)}{N} \cdot \sum (x) + N\frac{(\sum (x))^2}{N^2}$$

Simplifying:

$$SS = \sum (x^2) - \frac{2(\sum x)^2}{N} + \frac{(\sum x)^2}{N}$$

$$= \sum (x^2) - \frac{(\sum x)^2}{N}$$

$\sum (x)$ is the total of the x values $= T$,

$$\therefore SS = \sum (x^2) - \frac{T^2}{N}$$

And therefore the population variance estimate from a sample:

$$s^2 = \frac{\sum (x^2) - (T^2/N)}{N - 1}$$

The standard deviation of the population from a sample is:

$$s = \sqrt{\frac{\sum (x^2) - (T^2/N)}{N - 1}}$$

The advantage of this formula is that T, the total of the values, and $\sum (x^2)$, the total of the squared values, can both be accumulated on a calculating machine. Note that the use of this formula does not involve subtracting values from the mean, or even calculating the mean. Additional values can easily be added without lengthy recalculation.

APPENDIX 3. DETAILED WORKING OF HYPOTHETICAL EXAMPLES OF THE USE OF THE t TEST

Experiment 1

It is suggested that patients coming to afternoon surgery are more anxious than patients coming to morning surgery because of the longer period of waiting. Pre-operative pulse rates are obtained for two matched groups of eleven patients.

Group A—morning Pulse rates			Group B—afternoon Pulse rates		
(x)	$(x - \bar{x})$	$(x - \bar{x})^2$	(x')	$(x' - \bar{x}')$	$(x - \bar{x}')^2$
61	−13	169	69	−11	121
66	−8	64	64	−15	225
91	+17	289	95	+16	256
84	+10	100	92	+13	169
75	+1	1	76	−3	9
72	−2	4	80	+1	1
79	+5	25	88	+9	81
69	−5	25	69	−10	100
74	0	0	70	−9	81
71	−3	9	79	0	0
72	−2	4	88	+9	81
$\sum x = 814$	0	$SS_x = 690$	$\sum x' = 869$	0	$SS'_x = 1124$

Continued on next page

$$N = 11 \qquad\qquad N' = 11$$

$$\bar{x} = \frac{\Sigma x}{N} = \frac{814}{11} = 74/\text{min} \qquad \bar{x}' = \frac{\Sigma x'}{N'} = \frac{869}{11} = 79/\text{min}$$

$$\text{var}\,(x) = \frac{SS}{N} = \frac{690}{11} = 62{\cdot}7 \qquad \text{var}\,(x') = \frac{SS'}{N'} = \frac{1124}{11} = 102{\cdot}2$$

$$\text{S.D.}(x) = \sqrt{62{\cdot}7} = 7{\cdot}92 \qquad \text{S.D.}(x') = \sqrt{102{\cdot}2} = 10{\cdot}1$$

(The figures have been chosen to give easily managed whole numbers, so that the naturally derived formula for variance could be used as described on pages 258. In a sample of natural data it is almost always quicker and easier to obtain SS—the sum of squared deviations, using the formula of Appendix 2).

Both groups can be used to estimate the theoretical population variance, by dividing SS by $N - 1$:

$$s^2 = \frac{690}{10} = 69 \qquad \text{and} \qquad s'^2 = \frac{1124}{10} = 112{\cdot}4$$

The variance estimate derived from the afternoon cases is greater than that derived from the morning ones. Is this difference significant? It is possible to set up the hypothesis that the response to anxiety is very variable, and that this accounts for the larger variance. Alternatively, could random samples of eleven have variances such as these, quite by chance? Before we can go on to test for the significance of the difference between the mean pulse rates of the two groups, it is necessary to settle this point. This is tested by an F-test. The larger variance estimate is divided by the smaller:

$$F = \frac{112{\cdot}4}{69} = 1{\cdot}63$$

Reference to Table 2 of Statistical Tables with 10 degrees of freedom for each sample, shows that values of F greater than $2{\cdot}98$ occur less commonly than five times in a hundred (the table is constructed for $p = 0{\cdot}05$). We can assume, therefore, that our value of $1{\cdot}63$ could easily arise by chance, and that there is no significant difference between the two variances.

Having established that the variances are effectively the same, we can pool the two samples to obtain the *best estimate* of the population variance:

$$\text{(pooled) } s^2 = \frac{SS + SS'}{(N-1) + (N'-1)}$$

$$= \frac{690 + 1124}{10 + 10} = \frac{1814}{20} = \underline{90\cdot7}$$

The variance for each mean is found from the formula:

$$s_{\bar{x}}^2 = \frac{s^2}{N}$$

and the standard error for each mean can now be calculated if required:

$$s_{\bar{x}} = \sqrt{\frac{s^2}{N}} = \sqrt{\frac{90\cdot7}{11}} = \sqrt{8\cdot24} = 2\cdot87$$

t is computed from the formula:

$$t = \frac{|\bar{x} - \bar{x}'|}{s_{(\bar{x}-\bar{x}')}}$$

The numerator we can do easily, i.e.

$$|74 - 79| = \underline{5} \text{ (absolute)}$$

The denominator is the square root of the sum of the two sample mean variances:

$$s_{(\bar{x}-\bar{x}')} = \sqrt{\frac{s^2}{N} + \frac{s^2}{N'}}$$

As the samples are of equal size, this can be simplified to

$$s_{(\bar{x}-\bar{x}')} = \sqrt{\frac{2s^2}{N}} = \sqrt{\frac{2 \times 90\cdot7}{11}}$$

$$= \sqrt{16\cdot4} = \underline{4\cdot05}$$

Therefore

$$t = \frac{|\bar{x} - \bar{x}'|}{s_{(\bar{x}-\bar{x}')}} = \frac{5}{4\cdot05} = 1\cdot23$$

Looking up the critical values of t in Table 3 of the Statistical Tables at 20 DF, we find that t must exceed 2·09 for the difference to be significant at the 5 per cent level. We cannot reject the null hypothesis, therefore, and must accept that a mean difference of five could have occurred by chance.

Actually, our original hypothesis was that the afternoon patients would be more anxious and have a *higher* pulse rate. A one-tailed test is therefore appropriate, but even so the critical value (1·73) is not reached, and we cannot even assert that the second mean is significantly greater.

Note, that if our mean values had been based on a total of 220 values instead of about 20, the *SS* would have been about 20,000 instead of 2000 and the best estimate of the variance about

$$\frac{20000}{220} \simeq 90$$

i.e. almost the same. BUT the standard error of the difference would have been:

$$\sqrt{\frac{2 \times 90}{218}} = \sqrt{0.82} \simeq 0.9, \text{ instead of } 4.05$$

This would make

$$t \simeq \frac{5}{0.9} \simeq 5.5$$

which would be significant at the 1 per cent level. Our earlier result is not necessarily an indication that our hypothesis is valueless; it can be regarded as an indication to increase the numbers of cases in the trial. It also brings out the mathematical basis for the fact that we are more inclined to believe in the reality of a relatively small change in mean pulse rate, when the means are based on a large number rather than a small number.

Experiment 2

Suppose now that the same data apply to an experiment in which the x-values are pre-operative pulse rates in patients undergoing a first insertion of radium, and the x'-values are the pre-operative pulse rates of the same patients undergoing a second insertion of radium 1 week later. We would like to know whether there is any evidence that patients are more, or less anxious facing the second operation. This is a situation in which the differences between patients is not relevant, and only the difference in each patient between one occasion and another is of interest.

The first step is to derive these differences:

x	x'	$x - x' = d$	d^2
61	68	+7	14
66	64	−2	4
91	95	+4	16
84	92	+8	64
75	76	+1	1
72	80	+8	64
79	88	+9	81
69	69	0	0
74	70	−4	16
71	79	+8	64
72	88	+16	256
—	—	$\sum d = +55$	$\sum d^2 = 580$

$$N = 11$$

$$\bar{d} = \frac{\sum d}{N} = \frac{+55}{11} = +5$$

$$\text{var}(d) = \frac{\sum d^2}{N} = \frac{580}{11} = 52 \cdot 7$$

$$\text{S.D.}(d) = \sqrt{52 \cdot 7} = 7 \cdot 26$$

The next step is to estimate the variance of the theoretical population of differences from the sample of differences. (As there is only one sample of differences an F-test is neither possible nor necessary.)

$$s_d{}^2 = \frac{\sum d^2}{N-1} = \frac{580}{10} = 58$$

The standard error of the mean differences is the square root of the population variance divided by N.

$$s_{\bar{d}} = \sqrt{\frac{s_d{}^2}{N}} = \sqrt{\frac{58}{11}} = \sqrt{5 \cdot 27} = 2 \cdot 3$$

$$t = \frac{\bar{d}}{s_{\bar{d}}} = \frac{5}{2 \cdot 3} = 2 \cdot 17$$

Entering Table 3 of Statistical Tables with 10 DF (one less than the number of differences) the critical values for t are found to be $1 \cdot 81$ for one tail and $2 \cdot 23$ for both tails. In the experiment as planned, it was not possible to say whether the patients would be more or less anxious, and a two-tailed test should be used. The calculated value ($2 \cdot 17$) does not exceed the critical value ($2 \cdot 23$) and so the difference is not significant at the 5 per cent level.

However, as a result of the experiments it is now possible to suggest that the first experience of radium insertion is unpleasant, and that patients are likely to be more anxious the second time. The calculated figure of t exceeds the critical value for a one-tailed test, and one can say that there is a significant *increase* ($P < 0 \cdot 05$). However, it is a very marginal result, and the acquisition of further data would be wise.

In general, the hypotheses which underlie experiments most commonly imply an expectation of change in some measurement in a specified direction, and one-tailed tests are much more commonly correct than two-tailed tests.

APPENDIX 4. YATES CORRECTION

In computing chi-squared (χ^2) where there are only two categories, every difference between expectation and observations ($E - O$) is reduced by $0 \cdot 5$ units. This is then squared, and chi-squared computed as usual. If subtracting $0 \cdot 5$ reduces ($E - O$) to zero or a negative quantity, that term is eliminated from the computation.

APPENDIX 5. CALCULATION OF REGRESSION SLOPE (b)

$$b = \frac{\sum (x - \bar{x})(y - \bar{y})}{\sum (x - \bar{x})^2}$$

The numerator is called the *covariance* of x and y and can be designated SP_{xy} (sum of products). The denominator is familiar as SS_x (sum of squares). For machine computation the above formula can be redrawn as follows:

$$b = \frac{\sum xy - [(\sum x)(\sum y)/N]}{\sum x^2 - [(\sum x)^2/N]}$$

APPENDIX 6. THE ERROR VARIANCE

If $\tilde{y}$ is the 'true' value of y as given by the regression equation for each value of x, the error variance ($s_{y.x}^2$) is given by the formula

$$s_{y.x^2} = \frac{\sum (y - \tilde{y})^2}{N - 2}$$

Note, division by $N - 2$ makes $s_{y.x}^2$ an unbiased estimate of $\sigma_{y.x}^2$, just as division by $N - 1$, made s^2 (sample variance) an unbiased estimate of σ^2 (population variance). There are $N - 2$ degrees of freedom because two parameters are being estimated (mean *and* slope).

APPENDIX 7. CONFIDENCE INTERVAL FOR THE TRUE SLOPE (β)

$$\beta = b \pm t\left(\frac{s_{y.x}}{\sqrt{SS_x}}\right)$$

Where $s_{y.x}$ is the square root of the error variance ($s_{y.x}^2$) and $\sqrt{SS_x}$ is the square root of the sum of squared x deviations. t, being related to two parameters, has again, $N - 2$ DF.

APPENDIX 8. DIFFERENCE BETWEEN TWO SLOPES

$$t = \frac{b - b'}{s_{y \cdot x} \sqrt{\dfrac{1}{SS_x} + \dfrac{1}{SS_{x'}}}}$$

b and b' are the two slope estimates. A pooled error variance $(s_{y \cdot x})^2$ is computed by combining the data and dividing by $(N - 2) + (N' - 2)$. t has $(N - 2) + (N' - 2)$ DF.

APPENDIX 9. CORRELATION COEFFICIENT (r)

$$\frac{\text{regression } SS}{\text{total } SS} = \frac{[(x - \bar{x})(y - \bar{y})]^2}{\sum (x - \bar{x})^2 \cdot \sum (y - \bar{y})^2} = r^2$$

For easy machine computation this becomes

$$r^2 = \frac{\{\sum xy - [(\sum x)(\sum y)/N]\}^2}{\{\sum x^2 - [(\sum x)^2/N]\}\{\sum y^2 - [(\sum y)^2/N]\}}$$

'r' is the square root of this quantity.

Significance of the correlation coefficient

$$t = \sqrt{\frac{r^2(N - 2)}{1 - r^2}}$$

t is entered for $N - 2$ DF. If the tabulated value of t is exceeded, the slope is significant at the appropriate level of significance.

Statistical Tables

1. AREAS OF THE NORMAL CURVE

The probability (P) that the value of any observation will lie outside given limits is proportional to the area under the curve lying outside these limits. Values of x^* [where $x^* = (x - \mu)/\sigma$] are tabulated for various fractions of the total area. This area lies outside the interval $-x^*$ to $+x^*$ and is found by adding a P value in the left hand column to one in the top horizontal column e.g. $P = 0.47$ has an x^* value of 0.722. The limits which contain 95 per cent of the observations are those which exclude 5 per cent of the observations: these limits are given by $P = 0.05$ and the value of x^* is therefore 1.96. A value $> 1.96 \times \sigma$ accordingly has a probability of occurring less than 5 times in 100.

Since the means of large samples are distributed normally the table can also be used to predict the range within which any sample mean is likely to lie at any desired level of probability (*see* page 266). In this case $x^* = (\bar{x} - \mu)/\text{SEM}$ and 5 per cent of sample means lie outside the limits μ (population mean) $\pm 1.96 \times \text{SEM}$.

P	0·00	0·01	0·02	0·03	0·04	0·05	0·06	0·07	0·08	0·09
0·00	∞	2·58	2·33	2·17	2·05	1·96	1·88	1·82	1·75	1·70
0·10	1·64	1·60	1·55	1·51	1·48	1·44	1·41	1·37	1·34	1·31
0·20	1·28	1·25	1·23	1·20	1·17	1·15	1·13	1·10	1·08	1·06
0·30	1·04	1·02	0·994	0·974	0·954	0·935	0·915	0·896	0·878	0·860
0·40	0·842	0·824	0·806	0·789	0·772	0·755	0·739	0·722	0·706	0·690
0·50	0·674	0·659	0·643	0·628	0·613	0·598	0·583	0·568	0·553	0·539
0·60	0·524	0·510	0·496	0·482	0·468	0·454	0·440	0·426	0·412	0·399
0·70	0·385	0·372	0·358	0·345	0·332	0·319	0·305	0·292	0·279	0·266
0·80	0·253	0·240	0·228	0·215	0·202	0·189	0·176	0·164	0·151	0·138
0·90	0·126	0·113	0·100	0·0878	0·0753	0·0627	0·0502	0·0376	0·0251	0·0125

Since any given fractional area is equally divided between both tails of the curve, x^* corresponding to a particular area in one tail is found by entering the table at twice the desired value of P. Thus $P = 0.05$ in both tails at $x^* = 1.96$; but $P = 0.05$ in one tail when $P = 0.10$ in both tails, at $x^* = 1.64$. Likewise, $P = 0.01$ in both tails at $x^* = 2.58$, in one tail at $x^* = 2.33$.

2. THE F-DISTRIBUTION

The F-distribution arises when two independent *estimates* of a variance are divided one by the other. If the values in the Table are *exceeded* for the appropriate sample size, the variances are too dissimilar to have come from the same population (95 per cent probability*).

DF=1	2	3	4	5	6	7	8	10	12	24
DF' = 2	18·5	19·0	19·2	19·2	19·3	19·3	19·4	19·4	19·4	19·4	19·5
3	10·1	9·55	9·28	9·12	9·01	8·94	8·89	8·85	8·79	8·74	8·64
4	7·71	6·94	6·59	6·39	6·26	6·16	6·09	6·04	5·96	5·91	5·77
5	6·61	5·79	5·41	5·19	5·05	4·95	4·88	4·82	4·74	4·68	4·53
6	5·99	5·14	4·76	4·53	4·39	4·28	4·21	4·15	4·06	4·00	3·84
7	5·59	4·74	4·35	4·12	3·97	3·87	3·79	3·73	3·64	3·57	3·41
8	5·32	4·46	4·07	3·84	3·69	3·58	3·50	3·44	3·35	3·28	3·12
9	5·12	4·26	3·86	3·63	3·48	3·37	3·29	3·23	3·14	3·07	2·90
10	4·96	4·10	3·71	3·48	3·33	3·22	3·14	3·07	2·98	2·91	2·74
12	4·75	3·89	3·49	3·26	3·11	3·00	2·91	2·85	2·75	2·69	2·51
15	4·54	3·68	3·29	3·06	2·90	2·79	2·71	2·64	2·54	2·48	2·29
20	4·35	3·49	3·10	2·87	2·71	2·60	2·51	2·45	2·35	2·28	2·08
24	4·26	3·40	3·01	2·78	2·62	2·51	2·42	2·36	2·25	2·18	1·98
30	4·17	3·32	2·92	2·69	2·53	2·42	2·33	2·27	2·16	2·09	1·89
40	4·08	3·23	2·84	2·61	2·45	2·34	2·25	2·18	2·08	2·00	1·79
60	4·00	3·15	2·76	2·53	2·37	2·25	2·17	2·10	1·99	1·92	1·70

DF, and DF' are the degrees of freedom of numerator and denominator respectively.

* Another table would need to be consulted for 99 per cent probability.

3. THE T-DISTRIBUTION

If the values in the table are *exceeded* at the appropriate degrees of freedom, the result is significant at the stated level of probability.

Degrees of freedom	Two-tailed test		One-tailed test	
	$P = 0.05$	$P = 0.01$	$P = 0.05$	$P = 0.01$
1	12·7	63·7	6·31	31·82
2	4·30	9·93	2·92	6·70
3	3·18	5·84	2·35	4·54
4	2·78	4·60	2·13	3·75
5	2·57	4·03	2·02	3·37
6	2·45	3·71	1·94	3·14
7	2·36	3·50	1·90	3·00
8	2·31	3·36	1·86	2·90
9	2·26	3·25	1·83	2·82
10	2·23	3·17	1·81	2·76
12	2·18	3·05	1·78	2·68
15	2·13	2·95	1·75	2·60
20	2·09	2·85	1·73	2·53
25	2·06	2·79	1·71	2·49
30	2·04	2·75	1·70	2·46
40	2·02	2·70	1·68	2·42
60	2·00	2·66	1·67	2·39
120	1·98	2·62	1·66	2·36
∞	1·96	2·58	1·65	2·33

4. THE CHI-SQUARED DISTRIBUTION

This table gives the values of χ^2 which must be exceeded for a significant result at; $P = 0\cdot1$, $0\cdot05$, $0\cdot01$ and $0\cdot001$. The values of χ^2 are tabulated in degrees of freedom (one less than the number of categories).

Degrees of freedom	$P = 0\cdot1$	$P = 0\cdot05$	$P = 0\cdot01$	$P = 0\cdot001$
1	2·71	3·84	6·64	10·8
2	4·61	5·99	9·21	13·8
3	6·25	7·82	11·3	16·3
4	7·78	9·49	13·3	18·5
5	9·24	11·1	15·1	20·5
6	10·6	12·6	16·8	22·5
7	12·0	14·1	18·5	24·3
8	13·4	15·5	20·1	26·1
9	14·7	16·9	21·7	27·9
10	16·0	18·3	23·2	29·6
12	18·5	21·0	26·2	32·9
15	22·3	25·0	30·6	37·7
20	28·4	31·4	37·6	45·3
24	33·2	36·4	43·0	51·2
30	40·3	43·8	50·9	59·7
40	51·8	55·8	63·7	73·4
60	74·4	79·1	88·4	99·6

Index

311